Healing When It Seems Impossible

Healing When It Seems Impossible

7 Keys to Defy the Odds

Shiroko Sokitch, MD

with Tracy Friesen

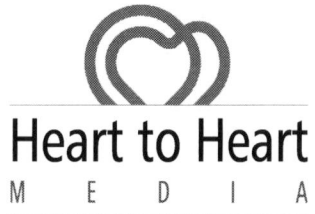

Heart to Heart
M E D I A

Heart to Heart Media™
Heart to Heart Medical Center
2200 Range Ave Ste 109
Santa Rosa, CA 95403

Copyright © 2018-2019 by Shiroko Sokitch, MD
www.HeartToHeartMedicalCenter.com

All rights reserved. No part of this book may be reproduced or transmitted in any form or by any means, electronic or mechanical, including photocopying, recordings, or by any information storage and retrieval system, without written permission from the author, except for the inclusion of a brief quotation in a review.

10 9 8 7 6 5 4 3
First Edition 2018
Second Edition 2019
Printed in the United States of America

ISBN: 978-0-692-18827-9
Library of Congress Control Number: 2018958896

Cover & book design by CenterPointe Media
www.CenterPointeMedia.com

Table of Contents

Dedication 9
Disclaimer 10
Acknowledgements 11
Foreword 13

Part I
The Miracle of Our Existence

Introduction
Defying the Odds 17

My Story: When Love Meets Medicine 26

What Does It Mean to Heal? 36

How to Use This Book 47

Part II
The 7 Keys

Chapter 1
1st Key: Love—Your Healing Superpower 61

Chapter 2
2nd Key: Physical Balance and Vitality 95

Chapter 3
3rd Key: Choosing Your Unique Lifestyle 128

Chapter 4
4th Key: Listening to Your Body 161

Chapter 5
5th Key: Emotions and Your Body 192

Chapter 6
6th Key: Never Give Up! Patience and Persistence 225

Chapter 7
7th Key: Trusting the Process 249

Table of Contents

Conclusion 281

Appendix A
Chinese Medicine 101: An Introduction 285

Appendix B
Lifestyle Suggestions 299

Appendix C
Resources 309

Index 313

Meet the Author
Dr. Shiroko Sokitch, MD, FMCP, DABMA 325

Healing When It Seems Impossible

This book is dedicated to all of my patients
that I've had the honor to work with over these many years.

Thank you for the love, strength and willingness you've shown
in seeking your healing.

Disclaimer

This book is not intended to take the place of medical advice or care of physicians. The reader should regularly consult a physician about matters relating to his/her health, particularly in relation to symptoms that may require diagnosis or medical attention. This book is not intended to take the place of consultation with a licensed medical professional.

The statements made in the book about products, treatments, and services have not been evaluated by the US Food and Drug Administration. Please consult with your own medical professional regarding the suggestions made in this book.

While all the stories detailed in this book are true, names and circumstances were changed to protect the identity of the actual patient.

Except as specifically stated in this book, neither the author or publisher, or any other authors, contributors, or other representatives will be liable for damages arising out of or in connection with the use of this book. This is a comprehensive limitation of liability that applies to all damages of any kind including (without limitation) compensatory, direct, indirect, or consequential damages: loss of data, loss of or damage to property, and claims of third parties.

Acknowledgements

First of all, I want to acknowledge my dear friend and soul sister, Tracy Friesen, who has poured her heart and soul into this project, and without whom this book would not exist. She has dedicated herself to helping me with the writing, the editing, and with every aspect of this book. THANK YOU Tracy!!

This book is my life's work. In so many ways, I've been living what is written here since I was five years old, and so many people have helped me arrive at this place.

Sivan Garr—thank you for your beautiful enduring friendship, love, support, guidance, and amazing feedback throughout the writing of this book. My very precious family of friends, who have been with me for so many years—your love and support has been instrumental in my survival and healing. Allison Massari—your coaching has helped me feel grounded in my messaging. Julie Clayton—your insightful editing work was essential in honing the message. Reynette Hong—my office manager and another soul sister—without you I would not be able to do my work. Dr. Anna Cabeca—you are an inspiration, a model of grace and compassion, and a brilliant physician and entrepreneur. Dr. Izabella Wentz—your friendship and support of my online presence has been incredible. JJ Virgin, creator of the fabulous Mindshare Summit and coach—I've learned so much from you. Members from my mastermind—I love you all and have deeply appreciated your feedback and input throughout this process.

Thank you to each and every person who has ever been involved in my life. Without you, I would not be here.

~~ Foreword

It is truly an honor to introduce this unique book to you. Only Dr. Shiroko Sokitch could have written it, as she lovingly guides you into healing no matter what it is you're facing in life, physically, mentally, spiritually and relationally.

Through this book, Dr. Shiroko helps us understand that we are not alone when we feel despair, fear, pain, anguish or a sense of loss. Through the 7 Keys, Dr. Shiroko weaves wondrous stories, real life examples and palpable solutions that take into account modalities of healing without discrimination. She takes us into seemingly impossible scenarios, and transforms them into *"it is possible"*. She uses her unique blend of Western medicine, Chinese medicine, Functional medicine and a true heart of loving devotion, in order to end suffering and bring healing.

As I read through this book, I was thinking of Dr. Shiroko reading it to me, sometimes with tea, sometimes standing in front of me, sometimes pouring forth scientific knowledge, but always full of all her love.

I do admit, when she first told me the order for the 7 Keys, I was quick to think that we have to flip these around—to start with trusting the process and end with love. As I read through the book, I realized it was the perfect order: everything begins and ends with love, which leads us to ultimately trust the process and ourselves … and leads us back to love.

The most powerful hormone, and my favorite hormone, ͞ activated when we feel love, and it is what strengthens us. Th.

us onto the right road and in the right direction. The 2nd Key empowers our physical self and addresses how every part is connected. The 3rd Key is Dr. Shiroko's insightful guide to choosing a lifestyle that truly works for our individual needs. The 4th Key teaches us the skills to tune in and listen to our body, which enables us to uncover its mysteries. The 5th Key is recognizing the significance of emotions in the body by making the connection between our emotions and how they physically communicate with us. This brings us deeply and fully into the person we are meant to be, healing our foundations. The 6th Key is practicing patience and persistence … and then some. With her guidance and love leading us into the 7th Key, we learn to trust the process and be okay with our body, no matter what we are experiencing. Throughout the 7 Keys, we are invited to celebrate who we are, and how we were made as we live this life.

You've been brought to this book out of curiosity, out of desperation and with an inkling of hope. You are holding a treasure map to discovering you. With this book as your guide and inspiration, and in the loving hands of a very skilled physician, healer and sage, your healing is assured. There is hope. Your healing is not impossible, *it is possible to heal.*

—Dr. Anna Cabeca
DO, FACOG, ABAARM, ABoIM

PART I

THE MIRACLE OF OUR EXISTENCE

Healing When It Seems Impossible

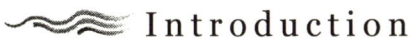 Introduction

Defying the Odds

"It is only courage on the path itself that makes the path appear."
—Paolo Coelho

Miracles

When I first began my medical studies, I was in awe. The more I learned about the human body, the more I realized that our very existence is a miracle. There is no other way to explain the brilliance of our design: the flexibility, the strength, the delicacy, the precision, and the capability of everybody is mind-boggling. When they are functioning well, it's like a concert—a symphony within—that is beautiful and perfectly aligned. As I learned what could go wrong with the body, I was even more amazed by the fact that we are all living, breathing, and existing—every moment of every day. Life itself is miraculous!

I grew up wanting to save lives. It was a strong and singular drive, and I had dedicated all of my life's energy to this one purpose. In medical school, I opted to become a surgeon because I thought it would be the best and most dramatic way to save lives and help people. But during my surgical residency, just as I was beginning my career as a doctor, I began to see there was so much more to saving a life than I had initially understood. Even when we, as doctors, saved lives, there was usually still so much physical, emotional, and mental pain that the patient needed to overcome in order to heal.

I quickly learned that my role as a physician was to address symptoms and try to alleviate pain as quickly and cost effectively as possible. The concept of "healing" was not a part of the equation: we sent our patients *home* to do their healing. In spite of my years of schooling, and so much technology and science backing me, I ultimately realized that I couldn't save everyone, and I couldn't help some people eliminate their pain. Sometimes the odds to truly heal seemed overwhelming.

I realized then, as a young doctor, that even more than saving lives, I wanted to find a way to help people *heal*. This passionate desire set me on a path to find answers—answers to questions that, at first, seemed impossible.

Finding Answers to Heal

Alicia was constantly ill. She had no energy, her body ached all over, she was nauseated every morning, had a headache every day, and suffered from chronic anxiety. She could barely get out of bed, let alone do what it took to raise her two kids with her husband and meet the demands of her stressful job. She had been to five doctors and had many tests, but everyone told her there was "nothing wrong." Several times she'd been offered antidepressants.

By the time she came to my office, she was on work disability and unable to care for her family. She spent most of her days in bed. Her husband didn't know what to do, and she didn't understand why this was happening to her. She told me that some days she felt so discouraged that she wished she could die.

A series of blood and urine tests revealed that she had an autoimmune disease, hormone imbalances, and several chronic viral infections. Alicia's baseline tests were in the normal range, so her doctors hadn't been alerted to these issues. We peeled back the layers of disease and rebuilt layers of wellness. Healing her body took a year.

While sometimes it seemed that she might never feel better, her health slowly began to improve, and she realized that she had been overdoing it for years. She

Introduction—Defying the Odds

had never really allowed herself to take care of her body and her own needs, and had always felt guilty when it came to taking care of herself. She wouldn't even allow herself to spend money on new clothes.

During Alicia's healing process, she realized how precious her life was, and saw that if she cared for herself, she was better equipped to enjoy and care for her family. Before her illness, Alicia's whole life was about duty and responsibility. As she healed, she began to devote more time to relaxation, spending time with her loved ones, and taking pleasure in her life. As she healed her body, her whole life changed.

HEALING WHEN IT SEEMS IMPOSSIBLE

This true story of one of my patients is one of many similar stories that I've heard during my more than 30 years of treating people. For many of my patients I am the "end of the line" because my healing approach and methods are "out-of-the box." My patients have complex health concerns, generally with one or more ongoing symptoms that seem to defy diagnosis or resolution. Typically, before they land at my doorstep they've already seen several doctors, had numerous diagnostic tests, taken various medications, tried supplements and other alternative methods, and still cannot find the cause or the cure for their issues. They are facing what seems an impossible challenge: struggling to manage day-to-day life with symptoms that drain them of their energy and cause extreme physical discomfort. They are desperate for some relief.

Maybe you, too, have migraines? Or maybe you suffer chronic back pain, or struggle with recurring anxiety, fatigue, or ongoing digestive problems? Or, maybe a little of each? Where do *you* go to find solutions? How do you heal when you don't know *exactly* what's wrong?

I don't have a magic wand or a secret code, but my experience as a doctor—having worked for 10 years in an emergency room and more than 25 years as a Chinese medicine practitioner—and also as a human with my own health concerns, has given me a unique perspective on illness and approaches to healing. When I work with patients, our journey together is a partnership. Together we can make a path toward healing, even when it seems impossible.

Together, we can walk *you* toward your own healing and wellness—beyond what you've even imagined. When you've struggled for a long time with your health, you may feel hopeless, or you may feel like healing won't happen, but I can assure you, just like the thousands of people I've helped in my career, you too *can* heal—even when it seems to be against all the odds.

I have faith in your body's intelligence and its capacity to heal. I've seen "miracles" too many times to think they are flukes or anomalies. I've come to realize that our biggest job, when we are healing, is to uncover what might be preventing us from getting to the miraculous.

Your body is your friend, and *it is designed to heal.* Part of our purpose as humans is to learn how to be hopeful when we despair, how to love when we feel fearful, how to keep going when we want to give up, and how to heal when we become sick. Through this life-long learning process—which is heroic and transformational—your body is your greatest school.

You may not believe it right now, but *your body is on your side!*

The truth is, healing and wellness are so much more than "standard protocol" and pills. Imagine if there was only one diet to lose weight, or if everyone needed the same amount of sleep at night, or even if we all had to use the same shampoo? Every person, every body, and every health issue is unique and needs to be approached individually.

Healing and being healthy over the long haul requires a balance between acting upon what we know (*i.e.,* practical science), honoring the infinite mysteries within your body, and good old-fashioned caring. This kind of caring is not just between the practitioner and the patient: It's about how you care for yourself, for your life, and for others.

When you feel that you are cared for, and that you care about others, caring becomes a way of life. Then, you feel supported, able, and willing to

Introduction—Defying the Odds

do the things that need to be done in order to heal.

INTRODUCTION TO CHINESE MEDICINE

When I first read about Traditional Chinese Medicine (TCM) and acupuncture during my second year of surgical residency, it felt like coming home. This 5000-year-old, intricate, highly developed, tested and proven medicine explains that our bodies are made up of energy, and this energy flows through our bodies in certain patterns. When our energy is out of balance, we have problems and become ill. Chinese medicine is the art of working with the energy in the body to bring about healing.

Energy is the foundation of *everything*, including our physical, mental, emotional, and spiritual makeup. According to Chinese medicine, every element of our lives—including our relationship with our environment, with each other, with our emotions, and with our spiritual selves—plays an important role in our physical health and healing. Therefore, health is all about relationship—how we relate to these different aspects of our lives. Chinese medicine teaches that everything in the body works together to create balance, so you cannot isolate one thing and expect the body to heal.

TCM explained to me the gaps that I was witnessing when a patient had an illness that didn't fit the standard treatments or diagnosis. Learning about this ancient medicine gave me answers to some of my deepest questions about healing. Of course, I never used Chinese medicine practices in the ER, but as I built my own practice, I learned to integrate different modalities rather than see them as competing theories. I now use them as building blocks to be arranged and rearranged to suit my patients' specific needs.

After decades of practice blending Chinese and Western medicine, I still love the magic that happens when the body begins to experience balance from within. So often it is the undefinable, mysterious aspects of our lives that are the most meaningful.

How Do We Heal?

I am a huge proponent of using all means available to address a problem. When a health issue is readily relieved through straightforward means, I am always thrilled. Medication, surgery, acupuncture, chiropractic work, diet, and lifestyle changes can all offer powerful and effective results. The challenge is when the issue is not easy to define or heal. When we keep peeling away the layers and not getting to the root cause, or when the standard treatment does not cure the problem, or when there is no diagnosis and nothing seems to help, we must ask ourselves—what else is going on? How do you heal when the answers aren't easy or obvious?

As I worked to develop a healing approach that could incorporate everything I had learned, I knew it could not be a standard formula. Every illness and every recovery is unique to each person, and so are the *remedies* that might work for each of us. There is no such thing as a cookie-cutter solution when it comes to your health and healing.

As my work progressed, I began to recognize that although there was no single solution, there were specific "keys" that facilitated healing in my patients. These keys offered answers—unlocking doors to the mysteries of healing. As they evolved, they eventually became the healing approach that I use with my patients, and that I now bring to you.

The *7 Keys to Defy the Odds* offer a healing approach that is fully grounded in the physical experience and integrates the holistic healing principles of Chinese medicine, the knowledge and remarkable advances of Western science, and the spiritual concepts of love and awareness. These Keys give you the tools to be able to live with your body, work with the particular elements of *your* life, and create a path to lasting health and wellness.

Introduction—Defying the Odds

> 1st Key: **Love—Your Healing Super Power**
> 2nd Key: **Physical Balance and Vitality**
> 3rd Key: **Choosing Your Unique Lifestyle**
> 4th Key: **Listening to Your Body**
> 5th Key: **Emotions and Your Body**
> 6th Key: **Never Give Up! Patience and Persistence**
> 7th Key: **Trusting the Process**

Healing is not just a physical process—it affects your whole being. This book is a roadmap to heal in a vital and fully integrated way. Through these chapters, you will learn to address your health on a physical, mental, emotional, and spiritual level in order to achieve whole healing.

Inside, you will find practical techniques and concepts that you can use every day. Each key offers real solutions *for you*, so that you can customize your wellness practice into your daily life.

There are countless books about how to change your lifestyle in order to heal, or how your mind and thoughts can bring you health, or how meditation and spiritual inquiry can create wellness—but it is *not just one thing* that makes us healthy. We can't solve the impossible with ideas that we've already tried … which is why it seems impossible! In order to defy the odds and heal, we need to use our imagination. It's means thinking so far outside the box that there is no box—because no box can contain *you*!

THIS BOOK IS FOR YOU!

Imagine the impact on your health if you truly understood your own body. Imagine if you believed wholeheartedly in your ability to heal, and if you had a deep sense that your body is your friend, and is constantly working on your behalf. Imagine if you no longer felt afraid of being sick.

Medicine and science are constantly evolving, but the goal is always the same: we want our health. We want to feel good. We want to understand what is happening to us, and when we can't understand it, we want to at least feel at peace. We want to know that we have the strength and the ability to handle what is in front of us, and we want the tools to be able to sculpt our future.

This book is especially written for you if you are facing a mystery in your body, or if you have a chronic or undiagnosed illness. And it is written for you if you are just plain tired of feeling bad.

There is a supernova of healing—and it's already inside of you. Your healing is already happening! The 7 Keys give you the instruments to unlock those doors inside of you and open yourself up to the life and the future that you desire.

Here's what you can expect on your journey to defy the odds using the 7 Keys:
- Improve your relationship with your body
- Increase your vitality
- Let go of your fear of illness
- Learn to listen to your body and understand its signals
- Find the root cause of your health issues
- Reduce stress, pain, and inflammation
- Regain your ability to get well
- Learn to filter through the massive information available and determine the right lifestyle for you
- Gain tools to navigate and release your emotions so they don't become stuck in your body
- Increase joy, balance, and hope in your life
- Fall in love with your body and your life
- Heal when it seems impossible!

Introduction—Defying the Odds

The journey to heal and be healthy, and to fully embrace and live every moment of your life is an incredible, heroic adventure, and *it is possible*. My intention with this book is to provide a renewal of hope, and to give you the experience of a miracle with your own health.

～ My Story: When Love Meets Medicine

"Healing begins and ends with love.
Love is the greatest healing force."
—Shiroko Sokitch, MD

OMA

I was raised in a small town in Germany and lived there until I was seven years old. My parents separated when I was three, and I didn't see my father again until I was in my twenties. My mother was in shock from the sudden separation, and overwhelmed by the need to take care of her children financially, so we went to live with her mother, my grandmother. My mom was single with two kids in a time and place where people didn't get divorced. She had to make money to support us, and her heart was broken, so she didn't have much time for me.

After we moved in with my grandma, my great-grandma, my Oma, became my best friend in the world. She lived on the same property as my grandma, but she had her own little house. I was always over there visiting with her and playing, and she was always happy to see me. She would spoil me—making me little dresses and buying me gifts. My childhood was far from idyllic, and my Oma was the one person who was always available to care for me. When I was in pain, she hugged and comforted me. I can still remember the patience and kindness in her face. I always felt her love.

My Story: When Love Meets Medicine

One evening, when I was five years old, I was visiting with my Oma and she suddenly collapsed on the floor. I was alone with her and didn't know what to do. I shook her and tried to wake her, but she wouldn't open her eyes. I raced to get my mom and grandma, calling, "Hurry! Come quickly! Something is wrong with Oma!" They came running to help her, but they couldn't wake her, either. They called an ambulance, and I remember the big stretcher being lifted out through her front room window because her door was too small.

A few days later, I was sitting outside my grandma's house on the steps, holding a stuffed Bambi that my Oma had given me. My mother sat down next to me, and through tears she told me that my Oma was dead. She said, "Her heart stopped beating; she won't be coming home anymore." In that moment, my whole world stopped.

Before the tears could well up in my eyes, I thought to myself, *there must be something that I could do to save her life!* My mind turned quickly, working hard on a solution. I imagined a machine that would bring my Oma's heart back to beating—something that I had no actual experience with, nor had I ever seen. With all my heart I believed that there *had* to be something that could make my Oma all better. I prayed for a miracle.

In that moment, the sorrow and loneliness that I felt was huge, but my hope was even bigger. It is my nature, and the nature of us all, to persevere. At five years old I did not understand the finality of death. I urgently held onto my belief that there had to be a way to save my Oma. The pain of this experience awakened in me a fierce desire to find a way to heal—*even when we are told there is no hope.*

That was the day I decided to become a doctor. That moment initiated inside of me a deep seeking, a calling, that set my life on a very specific trajectory. I was surrounded by pain and misery in my life and I didn't understand it. I wanted to make people feel better. *I* wanted to feel better. I didn't know anything about medicine or healing, I just knew that doctors had something to do with what happened to my Oma.

I had the sense, even as a young child, that there were answers no one could tell me. I had the feeling that life was so much more possible and so much more miraculous than what I was being shown. I didn't know anything about energy, but I could feel something bigger supporting me, and I wanted to be connected to *that*. From that moment forward, with tenacious vigor, I dedicated my life to understanding the body and the human condition on a physical level in order to help people *live*.

I was relentless in my pursuit, and everyone—my family and our neighbors—knew about my mission to become a doctor. I wanted to understand what was going on with each person, to learn how the body works, be able to overcome adversity, and survive against all odds. My dedication to finding answers was unwavering.

When I was 7, my mom married an American and we moved from Germany to Holland. Then, when I was 10, we moved to Washington state, outside of Seattle. When I received my first A in junior high, everyone was shocked. No one in my family had even graduated from high school, let alone considered going to college.

As I moved forward with my passion, it became more and more clear what was required: totality. Becoming a doctor requires sure-footed focus and determination, piles of money, ridiculously long hours, hard work, and endless schooling. As a woman going to medical school in the 80's, people were hesitant to believe in me, but my fire never failed. Like a heat-seeking missile, I was going to find and understand what it takes to heal.

Saving Lives

I will never forget the first time I helped save a person's life. It was a dark and stormy night ... literally.

I was a third-year medical student and it was my first shift in the Emergency Medicine rotation at Harborview, the County Hospital in Seattle. I was so terrified and excited that I could hardly breathe. I walked through the double doors leading into the ER and was immediately overwhelmed by the bright lights, noise, and staff who were busily running around at work. The resident in charge had no time to instruct me. He handed me the chart for my first patient and ran off to his next urgent task.

I was floundering, trying to figure out how to suture my drunk patient's eyelid, when suddenly I heard sirens and shouting in the hall. Someone yelled: "Gunshot wound! Three minutes out! Everyone to the trauma room, NOW!"

We all ran to the designated trauma room to prepare. The medics came rushing in with a man on a stretcher. There was blood all over him. One medic was giving him oxygen while another was holding a bleeding chest wound. As we transferred him to the ER gurney, eight people surrounded him—starting IV's, searching for other wounds, getting ready to take X-rays, and cutting off his clothing.

We found the hole in his heart and got him to the operating room within minutes. That night in the ER, I helped save a man's life! It was such a thrill! It was what I had been working toward all those years, and it felt absolutely miraculous. I wanted to do that forever. That experience is what made me decide to go into surgery.

As a surgeon, I thought I would be at the forefront of medical miracle-making. And in some ways, I was. There were definitely moments like that first one, when we would take someone from the brink of death and bring them back to life.

But as I spent more time with patients during my residency, I began to see that there was so much more to saving a life than getting the blood circulating again.

Residency life was busy; we were trained to remain professional, detached, and unemotional as we handled critical life-saving details. I found it difficult to stay connected to the significance of my work and to the miracle of saving lives. I began to lose my perspective and spent all my time and energy focusing on the task at hand.

As I worked and studied, I became acutely aware of the limitations of medicine. I had patients in excruciating pain, patients in the burn unit who were begging for relief, and there was little that I could do. I had patients who had been diagnosed with a terminal illness and who would look at me and ask, "What do I do now?" I didn't have the answers.

There were so many problems I simply could not solve. I was deeply frustrated, to the point that I began to question my path. After so many years of hard work and determination, my dream of saving people began to seem impossible.

Part of my drive to become a doctor resided in my insistent belief in miracles, and my desire to help make them happen. I wanted to get rid of pain—both my own and others'. I wanted to find a way to soothe pain, to remove it, and to shield it from happening. But as my studies advanced, it seemed that the problems and the pain were so much bigger than I had understood.

As I studied, and practiced, and learned how to save lives, I realized that *living was the challenge*, not the moment when death was conquered. Saving a life was not the end of the line; it was merely the beginning. Living life, handling pain, and finding a way to be peaceful inside it all—that was what I was truly seeking. But no one taught that in medical school, and I had no idea how to find those answers. I had dedicated every ounce of my energy, my mind, my money, and my time to becoming a doctor, and as I began to understand that achieving my goal was not going to solve all my problems, I began to feel like everything was slipping away.

It was at this time that I came up against some of my own personal issues. All of my focus and energy had gone into achieving my dream of becoming a doctor, so, not surprisingly, the issues in my own life that were out of balance began to show up. My unresolved childhood traumas began to affect me, and, coupled with my loss of professional purpose, I began to sink into a debilitating depression.

When I found myself wanting to drive my car off a bridge one night, I realized that I could not help others while I was in this emotional and mental state. I knew I needed to do something drastic.

THE NEXT STEP

I went to see a counselor. She suggested that I take some time off from work and connect with what I really needed. I was working 100 hours a week and had very little time to try to sort things out and heal myself.

My surgical chief reluctantly gave me a month off without pay. With no clear plan, I drove from Washington, where I was in residency, to visit my mom in California, where she had moved a few years earlier.

As soon as I arrived, I became extremely ill. I had a high fever, a severe headache, and I was so achy in my body that I couldn't move for several days. My mom had the wisdom to leave me alone in a dark room, bringing me water and broth when I needed it.

On the fifth day of my illness, I experienced something that changed my life forever. I was still feverish, floating in and out of sleep, and I had this moment that felt like a dream, but was completely lucid. I heard the words: "If you stay in surgery, you will die." As soon as I heard this, I knew the truth of it. When I woke up the next morning my fever had broken and I knew I was going to leave my surgical residency.

At that time, I didn't realize this was my "healing crisis"—my call to become a true healer. From that day forward, it seemed that life was showing me, step by step, which way to go.

I knew I wanted to continue to help people heal, and yet, I felt that I wasn't helping them enough. I knew I wanted to save lives, but more than that, I wanted to find the tools that would *help people truly be alive*. I wanted to help people heal physically, but also emotionally and spiritually. I knew, even then, that this journey to heal others was going to also heal me.

I had no idea what was next for me. I decided to complete my second year of surgical residency and then practice emergency medicine until I knew what to do. A month later, while I was still working in my residency program, I was introduced to a book called *The Web That Has No Weaver*, by Ted Kaptchuk. It wonderfully describes how energy works, and takes into account the *mysteries of life*. This book made healing sound beautiful. It was the first time I had heard of acupuncture. At that time, in 1986, acupuncture was a recent arrival to the U.S., and had never been presented in my medical training,

As soon as I began reading, I fell in love with the concept of Chinese medicine. I knew I had found my path. I was ready to move, to find Ted Kaptchuk and learn from him. Instead, I found the one person in our hospital system that practiced acupuncture, and he became my mentor. I also found a Chinese medicine school in Washington where I could study. I continued to work in the ER as I learned acupuncture, and my knowledge and appreciation of both Chinese and Western medicine grew in tandem.

After finishing acupuncture school, I had the dream of opening an integrative medical center, one where the best of both worlds could come together. I decided to leave Seattle and move to California. It took some time, but after two years I had found the people who would support my dream of opening an integrative center. In 1993 we opened Heart to Heart Medical Center in Santa Rosa.

At Heart to Heart, I was able to combine the science and advancements in Western medicine with the knowledge and understanding of Chinese medicine, to build a new way of approaching health and wellness. I realized that these two approaches, though dichotomous in method and philosophy, can wonderfully complement each other, and their integration can result in a much surer path toward healing.

As I built my practice, I learned more every day. I got married, and together, my husband and I grew my practice as partners. It wasn't all smooth sailing, but even with the turbulence, my life continued to move in a certain direction. My belief in the miraculous flourished and was ever-present because my life continued to feel miraculous.

THE MISSING PIECE
I believe that when we decide to learn something life helps us, and we go through whatever it takes to learn it. Usually, this process looks entirely different than what we might imagine at the beginning, and very often it's not what we think we want. But in the end, upon deeper inspection, we can always find those places and moments when we received *exactly* what our heart was seeking.

After years of building my practice and achieving so many of my goals and dreams, I still found myself searching. I still felt that there was more I needed to do; more that I could learn.

Chinese medicine had offered so many solutions, but there were still questions I could not answer. My hunger to find answers, help heal people completely, and take away pain had not receded. In truth, after years of practice, my desire to learn the keys to healing was stronger than ever.

Ironically, the event that initiated my deepest transformation as a healer *and as an individual* was something that I initially thought was going to destroy me. I had spent years learning about energy, becoming aware of how it travels and works and behaves, and somehow I thought that this knowledge would protect me. I thought that with knowledge and understanding, I could rise above pain. It was shocking to realize that my dedication to my growth could not protect me from the pain of heartbreak. My knowledge could not act as a shield.

When my marriage of 15 years ended, I learned something completely unexpected: I learned how to love.

The end of my marriage had me re-evaluating everything, and at first I came up empty. I plummeted into the deepest darkness of my life. Suddenly, I wasn't OK at all. I questioned everything. I no longer knew who I was in the world. I had been to this place before, this place of deep and unavoidable devastation, but it felt even more obliterating this time.

I had built my whole life *with* my husband: my practice, my livelihood, my happiness—even my belief system had become entwined in my relationship. When we split, I felt I had failed as a human being. I completely lost my center. I didn't know what I had to offer as a healer, a physician, or a friend. I lost faith in my ability to connect with people on any level. I was so angry at life, because I felt that it had taken away my heart, my love. Everyday miracles disappeared. In the midst of my pain, I could not remember that on the other side lay transformation and renewal.

I saw how fear had been running my life. When I was young, I was afraid of everything. Becoming a doctor literally gave me a white coat—a way to interact and help people, and to not feel completely helpless. But the white coat also created a distance—a shield that I thought could protect me from the pain I saw and experienced all around me, and perhaps from my own pain, too.

Finally, after months and even years of searching for my own healing, I realized that I *want* to love. I *want* to be a loving human being. And I can't be passive about it. I have to *fight* for my love. I have to stand up for my spirit. The pain I was feeling, the sense of betrayal, the heartbreak, the desolation—all of those things actually extracted my desire to love compassionately and wholly.

My dedication to being a loving human being was the only thing that brought me solace. It was the only thing that made me feel better. The totality of my heartache forced me to find and resurrect a deeper love inside myself.

I was blessed to have an amazing support system, friends who never gave up on me, and who believed in me even when I could not believe in myself. And I was blessed to have the strength of my heart. Even in this darkness, my heart continued its relentless pursuit to heal. I felt deeply humbled.

My Story: When Love Meets Medicine

The end of my marriage taught me that I am not supposed to be separate. All of my hard-earned knowledge could not act as a shield. My purpose—*our purpose as humans*—is to remain connected to life, even to the parts that hurt.

Slowly, as I tended and nurtured and gathered the broken pieces of my heart, I began to understand that the only thing that could heal the deepest pains inside of me was love. I needed to make my love bigger than my pain. I saw then that healing begins and ends with love. Love is the greatest healing force. Every question that I asked could be answered, and every moment of my life found meaning through love.

We learn from pain, but we heal through love.

My five-year-old self set out upon a journey to find answers and connect to the miraculous. I wanted to remove pain, and to save lives. My journey was far from predictable, but the process taught me so much! I learned how to navigate my own pain, and how to help others with theirs. I learned how to bring love into my work, and to help my patients see what is possible—even in impossible situations.

The purpose of this book is to help *you*. More than anything, my goal in writing this book is to help you heal, and feel supported, and not alone. My hope is to provide answers, or at least clues to finding the answers you seek. What I have learned in all these years of working with patients who come to me with their last ember of hope, is that *there is always hope*.

What Does It Mean to Heal?

*"The wound is the place where the
Light enters you."*
—RUMI

MADELEINE

Madeleine came to see me with many seemingly unrelated physical issues. She had migraines, allergies, and chronic pain in her neck and shoulders. Before becoming my patient, she had undergone two major surgeries. When she was 31, she had a hysterectomy due to painful periods and severe heavy bleeding. When she was 40, she had her gallbladder removed due to gallstones. She also suffered from migraines and had knee problems.

Over the course of working with Maddy, she shared a great deal about her life. She was unhappy in her marriage and had been angry with her husband from the day they were married. His lack of attention made her feel that he didn't love her, but she didn't want to end their marriage because she said it would be difficult for their children. Her parents had gone through a sticky divorce when she was an early teen, and she blamed her mother and still felt angry for their split.

In Western medicine, most of Maddy's issues were seen as different problems with very different solutions. From the Chinese medicine perspective, all of her problems were connected to a liver imbalance.

What Does It Mean to Heal?

According to Chinese medicine, the liver regulates the emotion of anger, the need to get things done, menstrual cycles, the smooth flow of energy in your body, the ligaments and tendons, and it deals with stress. I could clearly see how all of Maddy's symptoms were connected to one another. Even her gallbladder removal was connected to her liver imbalance.

Madeleine was my patient for five years. During that time, I helped her heal her body by using Chinese herbs to balance her liver energy and balancing her hormones with bio-identical hormone replacement. I used acupuncture for her migraines, and also to support her emotionally. Acupuncture is amazing, because it not only addresses physical issues, it can also help to balance the emotions. If I had met Maddy earlier in her life, it's quite likely she could have avoided her surgeries. Through the process of working together, she began to recognize and channel her anger differently, and to feel better on every level.

While working with me, Maddy began singing and dancing—which she loved to do—as a way to release emotion. She also changed her eating habits and began to lose weight. She reached a place of feeling peaceful and accepting of her marriage and her husband; they even fell in love again, 21 years after being married.

THE ROOT OF HEALING

In the English language, *heal* and *holy* are derived from the same root: *old English haelen*. In the West, we view good health as a blessing and illness as a misfortune. When we are sick, we often feel that something *bad* is happening, as if the illness was an enemy with an agenda to harm us.

Chinese medicine views illness in a completely different manner. Rather than seeing it as something that is "bad" and trying to "fix it," Chinese medicine views illness as an imbalance in the body. Illness, by itself, is never the sole focus in Chinese medicine because illness is not really a separate "thing." It is simply an indicator of an imbalance in the bigger picture of your whole health. The work of the practitioner is to find where the imbalance originates, and to use different healing modalities to help remind the body how to return to balance.

So rather than focusing on and trying to fix the *problem*—like being given pain medication, which doesn't actually *solve* pain, or taking cholesterol medication, which may cause a plethora of other problems—Chinese medicine works to help make the energy in your body move smoothly. When the energy in your body is flowing, your organs are healthy and your body's innate healing ability can function at its optimal level. For Maddy, she learned to find more balance with her physical body and emotions over time. Healing for her was a journey of learning to listen to her body, tuning in to her symptoms, keeping her emotions clear, and finding more peace in herself.

You may wonder why Maddy was my patient for five years. Certainly I have many patients whose treatments are much shorter in duration, but healing is a journey. When I work with people, we build a relationship. Many of my patients may heal one aspect of their lives, but continue to come to me as other things show up. Together, we peel back the layers, like an onion.

It is perhaps rare these days to establish a long-term relationship with a healer who walks you through the process of healing and crafting a wellness lifestyle. But your health conditions didn't occur in isolation or in a single moment—they evolved over time, and similarly may resolve over time.

Once Maddy approached her health from a more integrative perspective, taking into account her emotions as well as her body, all of her physical symptoms could then be addressed at a deeper level—and eventually at their root cause. Symptoms shift when your relationship with your body, your emotions, your spirit, and the sum of all of your parts are in balance.

Understanding Energy: Qi & Chinese Medicine

The power and effectiveness of Chinese medicine offers insight into our ideas around healing, and what it means to heal. In order to have a clear picture of how Chinese medicine works, we have to first understand *energy*. In our day-to-day lives, we usually think of energy in regard to transferal of energy. Sometimes we have a lot of energy, sometimes we're tired and need to restore it. Certain foods give us energy, other foods deplete us. A fight with a loved one drains our energy, a loving interaction makes us feel more vital, more alive.

Chinese medicine says that our bodies are made up of energy, and that we are essentially energetic beings. The energy that gives us life is described as Qi (pronounced *chee*). Qi literally means breath—the air that is present in all living things—our life force, our vitality. It is what makes us who we are. *Qi* exists in rocks, rivers, bodies, light, computers; even thoughts and emotions have Qi. It is universal, flowing through all things, and in a constant state of flux. Learning how Qi works, moves, and affects us is the basis of Chinese medicine.

Thousands of years ago, Chinese medicine practitioners discovered natural patterns of Qi that travel through the body in channels or pathways called **meridians**. They identified 12 meridians that transport Qi everywhere in the body. It works like an energy distribution system. Each meridian is associated with a specific organ. Balanced Qi is essential to good health, so the work of Chinese medicine is to create and maintain balanced Qi in the body.

Harmony in the body sustains health on every level; when your energy is balanced and flowing, you feel good—you are healthy, not only physically, but also emotionally and spiritually. Illness is the product of blocked, disrupted, or unbalanced Qi within the meridians.

According to Chinese medicine, everyone is born with a certain amount of Qi, which we inherit from our parents at the moment of conception! We can also acquire Qi based upon how we live our lives. There are countless things in life that affect the flow of Qi. From our thoughts and emotions, to the way we sit at work, how we eat and exercise, to our daily interactions, everything that requires energy, (i.e., *everything*!) can affect the balance of Qi in our bodies … even how you arrange the furniture in your house. Chinese

Medicine practitioners work to regulate the circulation of Qi in the body through acupuncture, herbs, nutrition, and other modalities, adjusting the way that the energy moves, relieving imbalances, and impacting your health and life immeasurably.

Imagine that your body is an orchestra. When your body is functioning properly, it creates beautiful music and makes you feel good. Each "instrument" is vital to the symphony and affects the overall harmony of the music. If the clarinet is squeaking, the whole orchestra is affected. Similarly, if one thing is out of balance in your body, your entire body is affected. You cannot separate a symptom from the other parts of your body.

In an orchestra, if the squeaky clarinet is removed, there has to be a shift in the composition of the music in order to create the same sense of sound. If the composer and the orchestra are focused only on fixing the squeaky clarinet, the music will suffer. The problem needs to be addressed, but not at the cost of the whole. Your body, like an orchestra, works in concert, so that each part—your brain, your organs, the fuel you take in, your daily experiences—*everything* affects how the music sounds and how you feel at the end of the day.

OUR HEALING NATURE

Science shows that our body has a natural ability to heal—the information for healing is in our DNA and in each cell of our being. For example, when you cut yourself, your cells know that they need to divide and grow to fill in the wound. They know how to fight the infectious microbes that exist on your skin, and your DNA is replicated into each new cell that develops. Your body also knows how to gently turn off this process so you don't develop skin tumors. The best part is that this process is automatic: you don't have to mentally initiate healing. As long as you are alive, healing is possible.

We don't often think about this innate and miraculous ability to heal, but it serves us on a daily basis. Every illness has some mystery to it, and often,

What Does It Mean to Heal?

healing cannot be fully explained. This is why doctors and scientists continually seek new answers and solutions: there will always be more to discover. So, can there be a formula to heal? Is it reasonable to think that there could be a health method that encapsulates the incredible, dynamic, mystifying energy contained in our bodies?

And what does it mean to heal?

JOURNEY TO SOMETHING NEW

When patients first come to see me, they often tell me that they're sick of feeling awful and just want to go back to how they used to feel. We all have this hope or expectation that our bodies will always behave like a new car. We want to fill it with fuel and have it run smoothly for 100,000 miles without mechanical problems. We want our body to take us to and from work and allow us to enjoy life without difficulties. And when it does "break down," we want it fixed quickly and easily so our lives are not affected.

But here you are, reading a book called *Healing When it Seems Impossible: 7 Keys to Defy the Odds*. You've probably been dealing with a health issue for some time. For you, the "quick fix" hasn't worked. This may be hard to hear, but when you face a health issue that is challenging, mysterious, or chronic, there is no going back to the same person you were before. The difficulty itself changes you—which is what it's supposed to do! Your body is directing you to someplace new. Challenges are like sand in an oyster, causing the friction that creates the pearl.

In life, we see that adversity cultivates wisdom and strength, which ultimately improves our experience of life. When we face a challenge in our physical body, it's the same thing—it's an opportunity to grow on some level. We may not always understand why it's happening when it begins, but we can remember that it is there to help us.

For more than 30 years I've seen thousands of people go through extremely difficult times. I've also worked with a lot of issues in my own body.

During the hard times, when we are suffering, it always seems pointless ... and endless! But as the situation transforms and we begin to heal, we usually find that the experience has generated something new and positive within us.

> **Something amazing happens to every person who goes through a healing journey:**
> - You change physically.
> - Your awareness of your body becomes more acute.
> - You learn about the connection between your spirit, body, and emotions.
> - You experience your own strength and aliveness like never before.
> - You gain a deeper sense of gratitude for life.
> - You feel more compassion for yourself and for others.

This is what it means to heal, and this process is a powerful and heroic journey. Every moment, every step, has a purpose.

A MYSTERY ILLNESS

Tony is a 50-year-old man who came to see me after experiencing three months of severe illness. It started with crushing chest pain that came on suddenly one night. He thought he was having a heart attack. His wife took him to the emergency room and although all of the symptoms were classic for a heart attack, all of his tests were negative.

He developed a high fever, chills, body aches and a severe headache, so he was tested for infection and treated with antibiotics. None of the tests came back positive, and the antibiotics did not help. The symptoms were continuous and relentless. He was unable to function at home or work. Before all this started, Tony felt that he was a healthy and happy man.

What Does It Mean to Heal?

When Tony first came in to see me, he was barely able to sit in the chair in my waiting room. He told me that every day he suffered from crushing chest and back pain, and had severe headaches and night sweats. He was unable to sleep at all. It felt to me like he was carrying the weight of the world in his heart.

I did not have a Western diagnosis for Tony, but I knew I could help him. From the Chinese medicine point of view, he had fire in his heart. Fire, or heat in the body, is often caused by an infection, so I treated Tony with the specific idea that he had an infection, even though no tests gave that result. I used acupuncture and herbs to balance his hormones, nervous system, and immune system, and to help him heal.

After his first acupuncture treatment, he was able to sleep through the night. Within one month, he was able to go back to work part-time, and participate in family events. While his illness was never officially diagnosed, my treatment approach healed him. Tony went back to work after two months, and within one year he no longer had any mysterious symptoms. Today, Tony is completely healthy!

You may ask *why* this happened to Tony, and sometimes we may not know that answer. Usually, a difficult health issue that has no apparent "reason" is caused by some emotional or spiritual imbalance that the person is going through. It could be connected to past traumas—his childhood history, or stressful events in his current life. Tony and I never spoke in detail about "why" this happened to him. Thankfully, for him, Chinese medicine was able to resolve his issues.

I've found that we can't always answer *why* when the body goes through difficult times. Sometimes, we just have to trust that it's part of a necessary process for that person. This idea is covered in detail in the final Key: Trusting the Process.

"Healing" vs. "Curing"

To cure a disease means that you've found a way to make it go away for good. Our modern world is replete with chronic conditions that may never be "cured": Diabetes, hypertension, osteoporosis, ulcerative colitis, arthritis, chronic fatigue, and Lyme disease are just a few examples of issues with persistent, life-altering symptoms. *Yet it is possible to heal from these illnesses.*

Being diagnosed with a chronic illness does not have to mean a life of endless suffering. Healing is highly active, and dynamic. *It is a comprehensive change in the experience of your condition.* When you heal, you may still carry the diagnosis or some of the symptoms, but you are thriving in your life. You are well. Healing is not about the illness—*it's about the wellness.* It's about how to have the best quality of life no matter what.

It seems to me that *healing, rather than curing,* should be the goal for our modern health conditions.

Part of our understandable animosity toward illness stems from a notion that illness is the enemy. We are taught to be fearful, and that in order to survive we must fight. So we "fight" to lose weight. We "battle" a cold. We "beat" cancer. We "struggle" to be healthy, to exercise, to eat right, to sleep enough, and to live a balanced life. We feel, speak, and act as though we are at war, but in this war, we are both the enemy and the victim.

What if, instead, we understood that pain is an arrow, an indicator? Sometimes it is the flashing red lights and sirens that we need in order to adjust something inside of ourselves so that we can feel OK again. Symptoms can be a puzzle, and solving the puzzle means asking the right questions.

We ask: *"Why is this happening to me?"* and *"When is this going to be over?"* Instead, we can ask: *"What is my body trying to tell me?" "What could I do that might make me feel better?"* When your body is speaking to you, it might be the beginning of a journey.

What Does It Mean to Heal?

Transcendence of Suffering

"In some ways, suffering ceases to be suffering at the moment it finds a meaning."
—Viktor Frankl

In Webster's dictionary, "to heal" means:
- *to make whole or restore to wholeness.*
- *to bring something to an end or to conclusion, to settle, or to reconcile.*

The Western concept of health is deeply rooted in completion and wholeness. The idea is that once you heal, you are finished—as if healing is a static state. But as long as you are living you are constantly changing, and opportunities to heal come again and again throughout your life.

A study by Thomas Egnew, EdD LICSW, defined healing as *"the transcendence of suffering"* (Egnew, 2005). He interviewed renowned scientists, MDs, and psychiatrists with extensive experience with illness and death. His goal was to understand the common things physicians might be able to do that would facilitate holistic healing.

The study found that when patients feel their illness or suffering has meaning, and that they are learning and growing from it, they can achieve a sense of healing even when their illness is terminal. From this perspective, the goal of healing becomes finding meaning in our experiences, rather than alleviating external symptoms.

Healing Is More Than Physical

Often, when we are sick, we feel that we become our sickness, but *your symptoms do not have to define you.* I have patients who suffer incredible pain and still consider themselves healthy, and I have other patients who feel so weighed down by their symptoms that their illness becomes their whole world. Every illness and recovery is unique to each person, and no matter what you are experiencing, your journey to health is unique. Ultimately, no one but you can decide when you are healthy.

When I talk about healing, I'm talking about being able to live the life that you want. Yes, it's about feeling physically better, but it's more than that. Healing is not just physical. Healing means having passion, drive, purpose, love, connection, *and* the physical means to make your dreams happen. It means having a sense of wellness and goodness in your life. It means feeling more and more peace with whatever is happening—so that you can live your life in the best possible way.

How to Use This Book

"Only one who devotes himself to a cause with his whole strength and soul can be a true master. For this reason, mastery demands all of a person."
—ALBERT EINSTEIN

HEROIC HEALING

Joseph Campbell was a professor, writer, and mythologist who identified a classic archetype found in mythological stories across all time periods and cultures. He called it *The Hero's Journey*. I think it's the perfect analogy to our own healing journey.

The Hero's Journey begins with a *Call to Adventure*—a summoning toward an incredible goal. The Hero sets off from her ordinary life and ventures forth into an unknown world, where the path is uncharted, treacherous, and full of obstacles. The future is uncertain and throughout the journey, her doubts, fears, and vulnerabilities arise, but she always perseveres. In the end, the struggle is what shapes her. She becomes a Hero because she is challenged and she rises to the challenge. It is her strength, courage, heart, and grit that transform her from an ordinary person into a Hero.

I believe that when we become ill, especially with chronic, acute, or undiagnosed ailments, it is the beginning of a journey—a Call to Adventure. We are asked to dig deep and find inner resources to navigate what may seem like an impossible challenge. We are asked to go far beyond what we have already known. Our healing journey tests us, awakens our courage, and ignites our knowledge and understanding of ourselves. The goal is to thrive, and *the journey creates the healing.*

This book can act as a guide on your journey. Every Hero has a guide, a map, or a mentor that helps him reach his final goal. You can be the Hero of your own life! The possibility for healing exists within you. There is magic and mystery in life. With the help of this book, and by remaining steadfast in the pursuit of your goal, you will—even when you are facing an unexpected or impossible issue—find a way to put on your Hero's cape and become the champion.

YOUR GUIDE

Traversing through the 7 Keys that are described in the next seven chapters, you will learn tools to navigate, relieve, understand the body's pains, and accelerate your healing process. And, you will create a path of vitality and wellness that will last your whole life. Sometimes, you will need to seek the help of a professional to guide you on part of your journey; sometimes you will be able to do it on your own.

Each of the 7 Keys is broken down into certain foundational concepts, called **Fundamentals.** The Fundamentals provide the framework for each Key in each chapter. Each of the *Fundamentals* has corresponding actions that allow you to immediately incorporate the benefits of that Key into your everyday life.

You will also read actual patient stories from my years of practice. To preserve privacy, I have changed names and identifying characteristics, but all of the health details are intact and true. These stories illustrate the effect that each Key has had on individuals who have used them in their lives. They ground and give testimony to the importance and usefulness of the 7 Keys.

Chinese medicine is like the circulatory system of my practice—it runs through everything! In this book, I've taken the tremendous knowledge and ancient principles of Chinese Medicine and siphoned it into something that you can use in your day-to-day life. It is not designed to make you an expert in Chinese medicine, but you will learn some basic conceptual, anatomical, physiological, emotional, and spiritual principles that are found in Traditional Chinese medicine. This knowledge will give you greater understanding of your body, and why it is doing what it is doing.

If you would like to go deeper, you can also find more explanations and specific information in *Appendix A—Chinese Medicine 101* at the end of the book.

THE PRACTICE

The obvious and most systematic way to read this book is in a linear fashion, beginning at page one and ending at the end of the book. This is the order that I recommend, since each Key plays off the other Keys, and your knowledge will naturally build upon itself. Like a treasure hunt, information in one Key will lead you to the next.

At the same time, each Key can be understood on its own. Each is described individually, so if you really feel driven to focus on your lifestyle, for example, you can skip ahead to the 3rd Key. The best results, though, are achieved when you approach the 7 Keys from a holistic standpoint. If you focus on only one Key, you will see results in the other areas of your life, but like the holistic methodology of Chinese medicine, all of the Keys inter-relate.

The actions and activities that follow each fundamental will help you begin building your customized healing journey. These physical, emotional, and spiritual exercises can be incorporated immediately into your everyday life. Whether you read this book from front to back, or pick and choose the order, I recommend reading it slowly and implementing the actions as you go along to gain the best results.

It is also important to share your process with your health practitioners.

If you are receiving medical attention, you can share this book (or the ideas from it) with your doctor, acupuncturist, or healer. The more you and your healers can be on the same page, the greater your progress will be on your path.

SCIENCE AND INTUITION

Science has helped us make huge strides in healthcare and healing, especially in recent history. Just in the past 100 years we've advanced our ability to live longer, healthier lives, from an average of 46 years to more than 80 years life expectancy.

Medical science is a tremendous tool and it can be life-saving, but science is also limited in its scope. I have witnessed hundreds of previously held truths become obsolete as new science replaced the old. One example is when we thought that a low-fat diet lowered cholesterol. It used to be considered *fact* that reducing fat was the answer to lowering cholesterol, but we now know that *a low-fat, high-carbohydrate diet actually raises cholesterol.* Good fats are essential for brain, hormone, and immune system health.

Therefore, it is also important to learn to listen to your body and to apply your intuition. The mission of this book is for you to learn to integrate and incorporate both your intuition and what science has to offer.

This healing process is about learning. As you read and implement the practices inside this book, you will learn to walk the line between science and intuition so that you get the best of both worlds.

BUILDING STRENGTH

Before we get started, I'd like to take a moment and really look at the challenges we face when we are on a healing journey.

When you go on vacation and you miss your flight, or your luggage is lost, or it rains the whole week, you still enjoy yourself because you're committed to having a good time. It's easy to persevere when it comes to having fun. But when you're dealing with a physical ailment it's much harder to stay focused and keep on believing that it's all going to be OK.

I know that if your path to healing were easy, you probably wouldn't be reading this book. The challenge of a healing journey is that there are times when we *do* get stuck. We have moments—or days, or months even—when we lose our footing and start to think that we can't make our healing happen.

Remember: *You are the hero of your own life.* You have a goal, and you have the gift of healing inside of you. It is completely natural to have moments of discouragement, disappointment, and doubt—*that is part of the healing journey.* Through these challenges, we learn to face the difficulties, to show up, and to find something inside of ourselves that allows us to take the next step.

When we build our muscles, we first must tear them. That's what happens when you lift weights: you create damage to the muscle fibers in your body so that when you rest, the muscles repair themselves and build stronger muscles. In order for your muscles to grow, you must apply a greater tension to the body, a heavier weight than what your body is used to.

It's the same with all of our presumed weaknesses. In order to build our strength, it is necessary to experience our frailty and our flaws. We grow when we are pushed beyond what we have known before. Our faith grows when we experience our doubt and fear and find a way to move beyond them.

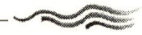

OVERCOMING OBSTACLES

There are certain classical obstacles on a healing path:

- Hopelessness—feeling that there is no solution, no answer
- Lack of faith in your ability to be whole again
- A sense of meaninglessness: "Why should I keep trying when I continue to feel bad?"
- Blame—someone or something is responsible for what you are experiencing
- Deep loneliness
- Doubts about the path you have chosen

Each of these feelings are valid, and even valuable. Finding the courage to remain steadfast and seek your goal no matter what is the quality of a Hero.

Below are some strategies to help shift your perspective when facing difficult challenges on your healing path. Oftentimes, success and healing is about finding the courage, tenacity, and strength to overcome the "impossible," to energize yourself when you feel depleted, and to "get unstuck" when you are bogged down on your path.

BEWARE OF INERTIA!

One of the most insidious obstacles to healing is inertia. It is borne out of a feeling of powerlessness and impotence, and it is insidious because it can act as if it is logical.

Inertia says:
What you're doing is not helping—you're still sick.
You can't affect the changes you want in your life, so why try?

You're tired. There's no point.
You're just going to be sick anyway.
You're getting old and there's nothing you can do about it.

And so on, and so forth …

Most diets, for example, only last two weeks. We lose interest, motivation, and determination almost immediately! Inertia steps in. Of course, we'd prefer our healing to happen fast and easy. The ideal would be to have it given to us!

Imagine that you are on a plane. When you take off, you feel the force of the plane; it pushes you into your seat. You see the trees and houses grow smaller and you are extremely aware of how quickly you are moving. But after surfacing above the clouds, the sun is shining, the sky is blue and seems to go on forever, and you almost feel as if you are not even moving! Your perspective has changed, but you're moving just as fast, even faster than when you first took off.

Those moments when we are above the clouds, or even inside the clouds, and it feels like nothing is happening … even in those moments you are moving quickly toward your healing. Don't give up. Don't lose faith. Don't become apathetic. Trust your path: it is leading you where you need to go.

GET CREATIVE!

"Any time you feel frustration, use it as a signal to get creative."
—SIVAN GARR

Very often, when we feel frustrated, we focus on the frustration. Instead, every time you feel like you've hit a dead end, or you're not getting what you want, inquire within: *"OK, how can I look at this differently? What do I need, right now, to feel better? What am I not seeing?"* Using your creativity in this way can help you find solutions, even with the restrictions that you may be facing due to your condition or illness. Move toward something that works and feels good to you.

Sometimes, when you've been dealing with the same issue for a long time, even creative problem solving can seem impossible, so you may need help. Find someone, a friend or a loved one, who is willing to be creative with you. You may just need a gentle nudge in a new direction.

FIND YOUR "YES!"

One of the most difficult challenges on a healing path is when we lose sight of our desire and willingness to continue when things are not going our way. Willingness drives us forward. One way to find your YES when you feel that you've lost it is to begin to look at your resistance. Begin by looking at your "No."

Here is a simple strategy to handle a lack of desire or willingness:
- First, look at the reasons *why* you might be resisting making changes in your life. Ask yourself these questions:
    - What is the benefit of your current situation?
    - What is your health condition preventing you from doing?
    - What is it allowing you to do?
    - How is that helpful to you right now? For example, perhaps you are tired of all the demands placed upon you, and being ill gives you the opportunity to say no. Perhaps you feel overwhelmed by your life at the moment and your symptoms are helping you slow down. You might not know the reason for your no, but asking yourself some of these questions might help you see more clearly.

- Next, look at the *benefits* of making the change—of going into the unknown, or continuing on your path—even when it is extremely difficult.
- Finally, after looking at both sides, take steps to move toward your YES. Move in the direction of your willingness and your desire to heal.

Remember to avoid self-blame. *Losing and then finding your "yes" is an important part of your healing.*

Practice Flexibility

We live in an ever-changing world, and your ability to move with the changes, to dance, to be flexible, is crucial to your healing. Keep an open mind when it comes to new ideas and foreign concepts. Try something new.

When things don't go exactly the way that you want, rather than becoming frustrated or disappointed, change your picture. Step outside the framework of what you think should happen. If you didn't have these ideas around the situation, what would life be like?

Develop your curiosity. Try doing something unexpected. If you can't stretch your mind about something, try stretching your body. Attend a yoga class. Get out of your comfort zone. Small or unusual actions can show your body that you are flexible and willing to change.

Remember, You Have Freedom!

You can choose your path toward healing. If you want to take medication and it will improve some aspect of your illness, take the medication. If you want to try different methods before taking the medication or having the surgery, talk to your doctor and see what your options are. It is your life and your body—you have the right to decide what is best for you!

Shake Things Up

If you reach one of those plateau moments on your path, rather than giving up or walking away from a particular course of action, try adding something new (and flavorful!) to your regime. Get your endorphins, those "feel-good" chemicals, going in your body.

For example, practice smiling, even if you don't feel like it. Exercise is great for releasing endorphins, so you could go jogging—but how about skipping, or hopping? Foods, including dark chocolate, strawberries, and spicy foods, and scents such as vanilla or lavender are also known to stimulate endorphins. Change your environment: try going out in nature. Wear clothes that you don't normally wear: dress up to go to the grocery store and see what happens!

Be Generous

When you feel poorly, it can be extremely difficult to feel you have anything to give, let alone the energy to do so. But there are simple things that you can do to open up a channel of giving and receiving inside of you.

Make it a point to smile at a stranger, every day. Bring a flower, or some chocolate, or a little gift to someone unexpected. Call a friend who you think might need some support. If all of that feels like too much, simply, and with intention, think kind, loving thoughts about someone in your life. Something magical happens when you do something generous for someone else, especially when you are feeling depleted or deprived.

What to Expect

The next 7 chapters are going to take you on a very deep journey to your own healing. The results may be surprising. It will be wild, tumultuous, miraculous, and beyond anything that you can imagine right now. Through it, you will find your own sense of healing, a healing that never ends. This healing process, this life, moves forward like a river.

How to Use This Book

You are ready for answers. You are ready to take command of your health and live a vibrant, full life that is brave and rooted in compassionate love.

Remember, your healing is already happening.

And, as with any good adventure, expect the unexpected.

Healing When It Seems Impossible

PART II

THE 7 KEYS

Healing When It Seems Impossible

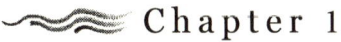 Chapter 1

1st Key: Love—Your Healing Superpower

"Love and compassion are necessities, not luxuries. Without them, humanity cannot survive."
—His Holiness, the 14th Dalai Lama

"The salvation of man is through love and in love."
—Viktor Frankl

What Is Love?

Have you ever noticed that when you're *in love*, everything feels good? Your body feels great. Emotionally, you can't be stopped. Even the usual stressors at work or at home don't get you down. It's almost as if love gives you *superpowers!* Whether it's romantic love, love for friends, love for a child, or even love for a stranger, our world feels brighter, happier, and more available to us when we are experiencing love. We feel alive!

If you think about it, every great mythical quest throughout time—from Homer's *Odyssey* to the story of Superman—begins and ends with love. Love flames our passion and our drive. It brings meaning into our lives. It is something you carry inside of you and can use at any moment, in any situation. So, it only makes sense that, as we embark upon our healing journey, we begin with the elemental, essential and transformative superpower of **love**.

Love is the greatest healing force in the universe. It is beyond an emotion.

It is a bond, an energy, an experience. In its purest form, love creates balance and unity.

Defining love can be tricky, because we all have different experiences of love and each of them is real. In the context of the 1st Key, Love is the *balancing and harmonious energy* inside of you that comes from your heart, from the center of your being. By its very nature—of being balancing and harmonious—love is *healing energy*.

When we allow love to color our worldview, it generates appreciation, kindness, empathy, and care. When we relate to the world around us with a focus on love, it changes our experience. It changes us. It can start with something as simple as trying to make the person in front of you happy, which generates warmth, laughter, positivity … essentially, love.

For so long in my life, I thought love existed outside of me. I thought I wouldn't be able to truly know love unless I felt it from someone else. Perhaps because of my upbringing, where I did not receive expressions of love, I was always searching to find *more love*, always looking for validation outside myself. Eventually, I came to realize that even when I experience love with someone else, it is *me experiencing the love*. The feelings I have are *mine*. Love exists inside of me, inside each of us, and it has the potential to be a limitless source of energy.

When we are in pain, or struggling, it can often feel like love has been taken away. The 1st Key helps us understand the limitless energy of love that exists within our own hearts, and the significant role it plays in healing.

A Healing Modality

When you think about it, our whole existence is about *relationships*. We are in relationships with each other, our body, our environment, our work, with our doctors and healers, *and* with the illness and the treatment we are using. All the different parts of our body work in relationship with all the other parts—including our blood, organs, limbs, and senses. Love can be seen as

1st Key: Love—Your Healing Superpower

the connecting force in all of our relationships, even the relationships within our own body.

I have spent years dedicated to working with energy and healing. After so many years, what I found is that the more I love, the better my patients feel. It seems that the energy of love makes healing more potent. So now, rather than focusing only on the more scientific dynamics of energy, I also focus on the energy of love itself.

You may wonder what it means to "focus on love". One of the fundamentals of this chapter is dedicated to exploring this idea and bringing it into your own life, but in a nutshell, when I focus on love in my work with my patients, I think about the energy of love, I feel it full inside of me, and I give it to them. My intention while I am working, is for my patients to feel better. I want the best for them. I want them to feel cared for—so I focus on those thoughts and feelings as well as the physical work I'm doing. This subtle change in focus shifts what I am able to achieve, and I have seen immediate results. Many people are experiencing dramatic change in just one visit.

ADAM

One of my patients, Adam, was in a very serious car accident before I met him. At 21 years old he was struck in his car by another vehicle and nearly died. He suffered multiple broken bones, a torn aorta, and a severe head injury. He spent two months in the hospital, most of that time in excruciating agony. Because of the aortic tear and the surgery he needed to save his life, some of the fractures he suffered couldn't be treated right away.

Adam was from a large, supportive family. He had five brothers and sisters who, along with his parents, rushed to his side after the accident, staying with him, holding his hand, offering their love as comfort to the relentless pain in his body.

Adam has told me that the love of his family was such a source of solace for him that it made his pain less intense. While he was recovering, he felt it as a direct and powerful healing force. While it couldn't take away the pain he endured, he knows that love from his family was what helped him survive the extreme trauma of his accident.

THE INTELLIGENCE OF THE HUMAN HEART

Scientists have shown that our heart, blood pressure, immune system, skin's ability to heal, DNA, brain chemistry, mood, and motivation are all much healthier when we feel love. The HeartMath Institute is a non-profit organization that studies, researches, and educates people about the powerful intelligence of the human heart. Their mission is to help people feel better by reducing stress and implementing techniques to self-regulate emotions and foster emotional flexibility. Their clinical studies have repeatedly demonstrated that feelings of appreciation, care, and love (what they call *"re-newing emotions"*) actually change our physiology, our community, and even the world. In fact, according to their findings, our individual experience of love actually can influence the earth's magnetic field!

On a more individual level, a study done at the HeartMath Institute showed that people who achieved a heart-centered, loving state and projected those feelings toward a strand of DNA in a test tube were actually able to alter the DNA structure! (McCrady, Atkinson, Tomasino, 2003)

We tend to think of DNA as relatively fixed, so this is convincing testimony about the profound and potentially healing power of love.

In other institutions, a 2005 study published in the "Archives of General Psychiatry" documented researchers who induced wounds of the same size, shape, and depth in couples. The wounds healed 40% faster in couples that were acting more loving toward one another than those who were hostile toward each other. (Kiecolt-Glaser, Lowing, et al, 2005)

Another study observed couples in which one partner had cancer and the other didn't. Each partner was put into a separate room, and the person without cancer was asked to send loving thoughts to their partner. The skin conductance of the sick person was measured, and showed a noticeable change during and even after the love was sent. Skin conductance is a way of measuring the electricity going through your skin when it receives certain stimuli. (Radin, Stone, et al, 2008)

Other research has shown that plants respond to love. So do water molecules!

These are just a few examples that show the veracity of love's ability to heal. Every part of our world is impacted when love comes into play. Beyond the science, we all know how it feels to be cared for—how we rest better, breathe easier, and just feel happier when another person has our best interest at heart.

These and other studies, and my own experiences with clients, tells me in no uncertain terms that the importance of love in our healing cannot, and should not, be underestimated.

Fundamentals of 1st Key
Love

In 1948, the World Health Organization defined health as *"physical, mental, and social well-being, and not simply the absence of infirmity."* According to this definition, feeling love is one of the most obvious ways we can feel good and be healthy.

The question is, how do we tap into the power and the sometimes elusive nature of love? And how do we expand it, and make it something we can find even in moments of stress or hardship?

The 1st Key is the cornerstone of all 7 Keys because it breathes life into the entire healing process. Love gives you the strength to move forward, to find answers, and to increase your belief in what is

> possible. Each of us has an endless reservoir of love-energy inside—which will deeply facilitate healing on this path.
>
> Below is a list of fundamentals that will help you build love as your foundation. Through a deep examination of these concepts, which includes descriptive patient stories and actions you can take at the end of each fundamental, you will learn how you can incorporate love into your healing process.

1st Fundamental: Your Body Is Your Friend

Your body is your ally, and it is constantly trying to communicate with you. When you are in a state of imbalance, physically or otherwise, this will eventually reveal itself through your physical being. Maintaining an attitude of loving friendship with your body and reducing the feelings of struggle or conflict that you have toward your health issues facilitates greater healing and eases your process.

2nd Fundamental: Focus on Love

When you see yourself as the Hero of your own Healing Journey, Love becomes your superpower—allowing you to do things that would otherwise be impossible. This fundamental teaches you how to keep your focus on love so you can improve your healing potential.

3rd Fundamental: Navigate Fear and Remove Blocks

Fear is our main block to experiencing love. There are specific scientific reasons why this is the case, and there are specific things you can do to navigate your body's fear response. When fear is running your life, and driving your decisions and behavior, it has gained too much of an upper hand. The goal is not to eliminate fear altogether; fear is necessary and useful in certain situations. You can, however, learn to turn your focus more toward a loving state—toward more expansion and possibility—even in the midst of crisis.

4th Fundamental: The Essence of Balance—Everything Is Connected!
Everything we experience in our lives affects us in every possible way, moment by moment and day to day. It's not just that one thing affects the next: every single chemical reaction inside of your body is precipitated by something else. Your body is in constant communication. Every cell and molecule is giving feedback all the time. When you consciously build your love, which has a tremendously balancing energy, love becomes a part of the communication loop in the body, and the ripple effect touches your whole body and life.

5th Fundamental: Community Support
The importance of having community and connections when you are sick cannot be underestimated. According to science, loneliness is as detrimental to health as love is good for us. Fortunately, when we become ill there is great potential to create community. People naturally gather together in a crisis—we want to help one another. Also, research shows that being vulnerable creates connection and intimacy, and when do we feel more vulnerable than when we are sick? Possibly the greatest gift of illness is in the connections that we make, and in learning to share our experiences with others and ask for help.

1st Fundamental
Your Body Is Your Friend

KITTY

When Kitty first came to me, she was miserable. She had been a physical fitness trainer for most of her life and was very health conscious, so when she was diagnosed with breast cancer at the age of 42, she felt totally betrayed by her body.

Kitty overcame the cancer through chemo and radiation, but afterward she felt tired and awful, and that's when she first came to see me. Her energy was low, she was fatigued, depressed, and she hated life. The cancer had been eradicated from her body, but the chemo and radiation had left her depleted and sickly. She was struggling financially, and not happy in any part of her life.

She told me that she felt like God hated her. She said she felt like she was being punished, but she wasn't sure what she had done to deserve such punishment. I treated Kitty with acupuncture and herbs, and as we worked together, she began to gain a deeper understanding and appreciation of her body. She told me that with acupuncture she was able to feel calmer and quieter. It gave her space to be able to be in touch with her body. Through that, she found her desire to be well again, and to love her body despite the physical pain and emotional betrayal that she had experienced.

She realized that even before she was diagnosed with cancer, she had been feeling an underlying anger at life. Her relationship with her mother had been fraught with a deep sense of betrayal. Kitty had always felt that her mother was not emotionally available and had prioritized her brother over her. As an adult, her fiancé, whom she had loved very much, had abandoned her a few years earlier. Wounded and angry, Kitty had not been in an intimate relationship in years.

Over the course of our work together, Kitty began to trust life again, and that was when she truly began to heal. And she blossomed! She ended up moving into a beautiful new home, her finances and business began to boom, and she eventually met a wonderful man to love.

ACTIVATE LOVE FOR YOUR BODY
How would I behave differently if my body were my best friend?

Whenever your physical self is giving you a hard time, it is ultimately helping you learn something—about yourself, your life, your beliefs, your emotions, your outlook, and so on. Imagine your body is your very own school. It is not trying to punish you or tell you that you've done something wrong; your body doesn't cast judgment. It is simply guiding you to find your healthiest self. Your body is like your teammate, a partner in your life.

For example, let's say you sprain your ankle. The message you receive from your body could be as simple as *"slow down"* or *"pay attention"*. If you have problems with your menstrual cycle, your body might be bringing your attention to your thoughts and feelings around your femininity. One of my patients suddenly began experiencing anxiety, and realized that she was desperately unhappy in her marriage. Her anxiety helped her see what was wrong and make a change.

When you work with a partner or friend toward a mutual goal, you make a commitment to listen, compromise, and work together to find out what the other person needs in order to feel good about the process. You also have to communicate your own needs and feel heard and appreciated. The relationship you have with your body is no different—it's all about listening and finding common ground. You may want to eat that delicious bear claw at your favorite bakery, but your body may not like it. Sometimes there can be a compromise, knowing the consequences. The important thing is to make decisions with clarity, intention, and care, and to consider your body as you would your best friend.

Taking care of your body can feel like a chore—something that is separate from the rest of your busy life. It takes work to care for your body, and it can so easily fall into disrepair. Sometimes we just don't want to deal. When we're young, this attitude might work because we're resilient, but as we age our bodies require greater and greater maintenance. Issues sneak up on us, and at some point this means we need to take more time to address and maintain wellness.

Fortunately, as you become better friends with your body, you may find that your attitude toward your health also changes dramatically. Eating healthy foods, exercising, and rest become simple and proactive ways to love your body and feel better. Rather than a chore, being healthy can be transformed into another beautiful, vital and loving relationship in your life.

Actions and Exercises for the 1st Fundamental
Your Body Is Your Friend

We've talked about how when you're in love, everything feels good. You can actually cultivate the feeling of being in love—inside of you. You can fall in love with your body, with your life. You can kindle the feelings of love that you have for your partner and friends. You can fall in love again!

The act of falling in love with your body requires sustained attention.

Below are some exercises that can help facilitate the process:

1. **Practice self-love every day.** Create a practice where you are showing love for yourself, and reminding yourself that you love your body. Each day, spend 3-10 minutes focusing on the love you have for your body. Here are a couple of examples of how you might do this:
    - Write a love letter to your body. For five minutes, write non-stop,

as quickly as you can, about all the reasons you love your body. Write down all of the things that your body does for you, all of the things that feel good to you. The practice of writing quickly and without stopping can help you access your subconscious. You may become aware of things you've never known before.
- Simply look in the mirror and tell yourself—"I love you. I love you. I love you" for 3-5 minutes each day.
- Make a ritual with your morning coffee or tea. Do each step of the process with love. Love the spoon and the mug that you are using. Give yourself a few moments each day and make the entire act an act of love for yourself and your life.

2. **When a part of your body is hurting:**
    - Rather than being angry with your body, put your hands on that place and ask what that part of you wants. Listen closely, as if you were talking with a small child who was telling you about her pain. See what you hear, or feel. What does your body need? What would make it feel more supported?
    - If you find that you can't be loving to the part of your body that hurts, find a spot on your body that feels good, and put your attention there. Let's say your left wrist hurts, but your right wrist doesn't. Examine the right wrist and look at all the ways that it's working for you, all the things that are right about it. Instead of focusing on what hurts, put your attention on what *is* working.
    - Pour love into the painful place on your body. Put your hands on it. Stroke it gently as if you were stroking a child's hair and hugging her. Love will help your body relax around the pain.
    - Do things that feel good physically, things that are about the five senses. Wear a soft scarf, have a tasty treat at lunch, light a beautiful candle, buy yourself some flowers, listen to your favorite

music, get a massage. Remind yourself about the good things about being in a body.

3. **Healing Is Your Goal**
    - When you are ill, shift your focus, again and again, to the notion that your body is working for you. Your body is on your side.
    - Create a mantra that reinforces this idea, such as, "My body is on my side."
    - Notice the moments when you feel your body is against you. Does that feeling come in moments when you are in more physical pain, or is it mostly an idea in your mind?

2nd Fundamental
Focus on Love

Love is your superpower. You have the ability to learn how to use it, to draw upon it, and to have it become an incredible healing tool.

My own experience with love is that it takes a fair amount of effort to stay in love, to come back to love, and to keep focused on love—especially when I'm sad or disappointed. Maintaining a loving heart does not specifically seem to be a natural thing. It takes work to get over your hurt feelings, to love even when you feel like you're not loved in return, and to focus on what is good when things are not going your way. But the effort toward loving *always* makes us feel better.

THE SEESAW EFFECT
Cortisol, which is released from the adrenal gland, is known as the "stress hormone." It is the body's natural, self-protective response to stressful situa-

tions and fuels our "fight or flight" response (also known as our fight, flight, or freeze response). When we feel threatened, cortisol is released and suppresses certain functions of the nervous system, such as aspects of digestion, immune system, and sexuality, so that all of our energy can be channeled into the brain and muscles and respond to the threat at hand. For these reasons, people who are under constant stress may have a weakened immune system, digestive problems, or low sex drive.

Our ancestors' stressors were very different than our own. They were running from predators, and the fight-or-flight response was ideal in those situations. In today's world, where we have an overabundance of stressors, our body responds to each threat as if it were a tiger, which means we may be producing more cortisol than our body needs.

Too much cortisol can accumulate in our system and cause inflammation and disease. Chronic inflammation (a side-effect of stress) contributes to cardiovascular disease, cancer, arthritis, and numerous other inflammation-based illnesses. It may also mean that you get sick more often, feel anxious, fatigued, or depressed, and can contribute to rapid aging.

So how do we "de-stress" in our over-stressed world?

On the other end of the hormone spectrum is oxytocin, also called "the love hormone." It is produced and secreted by the pituitary gland and it is an amazingly healing hormone. Oxytocin is associated with feelings of bonding, intimacy, and attachment. It is released when women are in labor and when they are breast feeding, and also during sex for both men and women. Oxytocin is released when we laugh, when we hug, and any time we do something that makes *someone else feel good*. It lowers high blood pressure, reduces anxiety, and strengthens the immune system.

These two hormones work together like a seesaw—so when oxytocin production goes up, cortisol production goes down (and vice versa). Therefore, oxytocin naturally reduces stress. The more you laugh, the more you play, the more you help others, the more you love and feel loved, the less stress you experience. This is a scientific fact!

The relationship between cortisol and oxytocin also explains the rose-colored glass effect you feel when you experience love. You feel happier, less stressed, more capable, and more connected to other people because you are experiencing the love hormone in your body—both when giving and receiving love.

Cortisol is not a bad thing—all of our hormones play an important role and we need them all to maintain balance. Problems arise, however, when hormones become stuck in "overdrive." Our daily life is plagued with stressors that don't kill us, but that our primitive brain perceives as life-endangering. Rather than being chased by lions and tigers and bears, we are chased by our obligations and expectations—getting dinner on the table, finishing that work project, making sure we're on time, dealing with traffic—all of which our adrenals view as insidious monsters and respond by producing cortisol. These "dangers" are not even remotely life threatening, but our body creates the same hormonal response as if our lives were threatened. The antidote is to balance stress with joy, laughter, fun, and love in our life.

Giving our attention and effort to the good stuff (or *love*) helps us begin to feel better. So treat yourself, and treat your friends and family. Make a point of doing something every day that makes you laugh! Laughter boosts immunity, decreases pain, lowers stress, relaxes your muscles, and helps prevent heart disease. Do things that make you feel good—make adult playdates, run around with your kids, have fun! By putting your attention on the sunny side, you will create more sunshine inside yourself.

ALIA

Before she came to see me, Alia already had undergone two minor surgeries to clear her cervical dysplasia. Each time it seemed to work, but a year after her second procedure, a Pap smear indicated some atypical endometrial cells, which could be a sign of uterine cancer. Her doctor wanted to do a biopsy to gather more information. Since Alia's body continued to struggle to clear the HPV virus that was causing the condition, her doctor told her that the best course of action might be to have a hysterectomy.

Alia had been having these issues for four years and wanted to see if there was something she could do differently to alter the outcome. She gave herself six months to try to heal her body before having the biopsy, and she came to see me. Together, we came up with a course of action.

Alia changed her diet dramatically, and I gave her supplements to support her immune system and her hormones. I used acupuncture to help balance her energy, which affected her both physically and emotionally. As we worked together she began to recognize that her shame and guilt around sex were influencing her sense of self-worth and her ability to love. She talked to her friends, received regular bodywork and acupuncture, wrote in her journal, spent time in nature, and prayed.

Six months later, her biopsy came back completely healthy and clear. Alia believes that love healed her. She told me that by focusing on her healing and with the help of my acupuncture treatments, she was able to open herself more to love—both within herself and around her. This created the transformation that she needed in her life on every level.

FOCUS ON LOVE

When you have been sick for a while and haven't found a way to resolve your illness, you can begin to feel that life is against you. It's not unusual to feel disappointed, frustrated, hopeless, and to feel betrayed by your body. This is especially true if you feel like you've done everything in your power to be healthy and strong. However, when you focus on *those feelings,* your options for healing are limited—hopelessness is a downward spiral. Instead, try building something phenomenal inside yourself. Shift your attention to loving thoughts, compassion, and understanding. It is already inside of you to become a beacon of love, light, strength, and healing. The actions and exercises below offer guidance to help you achieve this.

Something profound happens when you take an intentional step toward love—especially when you are in pain emotionally or physically. So often we focus on trying to get rid of pain rather than understanding the story behind it. Instead, send love to your pain. Imagine that you are healing. Imagine the place that hurts or feels broken inside of you is filled with light. Make a practice of focusing on the parts of your body and your life that feel good.

Sometimes feeling love is simply a decision. When your body hurts, it can be particularly difficult to access your love, but remember, *that moment is precisely when we need love the most!* Don't give up. Keep your focus on love.

THE POWER OF KINDNESS

A lot of the work I do with patients is to help them find ways to be OK despite the pain, symptoms, and uncertainty of not having a clearly defined diagnosis. One sure-fire way to feel better is through kindness.

The science of oxytocin says that it is activated mostly *in relationship*. Love itself is energy, so it makes sense that there is a flow of giving and receiving within the nature of love. Oxytocin, the "love hormone", is triggered when we do something kind for someone else (among other ways). But when you are sick, it can sometimes feel impossible to give, like you have no energy left to give. That's the beauty of love. With love, you don't have to physically *do* anything. With love, you can simply focus on your heart. Focus on the love inside of you. Allow it to expand. Send love to the world. Send love to yourself! Even when you are sick, you can do so many things inside of yourself that can open up that channel of giving and receiving.

Any time we are kind to another person, we feel better. Even when you're not feeling well, smiling at someone, or giving them a kind hello, opens your energy. Love acts like a boomerang: when you send it out to others, it comes right back to you.

1st Key: Love—Your Healing Superpower

Actions and Exercises for the 2nd Fundamental
Focus on Love

1. **Balance Your Heart**

   The HeartMath Institute studies the connection between the heart, brain and body. Their studies have shown that by focusing on your heart, you can balance your thoughts and emotions and attain more energy and mental clarity, as well as strengthen your ability to physically heal.

   Below is a technique developed by the HeartMath Institute to balance your heart rhythms so you can feel better. It's the perfect way to learn to focus on love! They call this process "Coherence". This simple practice can bring harmony to your body, mind, and heart. Try it!
   - Begin by taking slow, deep breaths. Put your attention on the center of your chest, where your heart is. Imagine that your breath is flowing in and out of your heart area.
   - Then, focus on a "regenerative" feeling, like appreciation, calmness, or care. Try to re-experience the feelings you have when you are with someone you love, or visiting your favorite place.

2. **Shift Your Focus!**

   Every time you catch yourself having a negative thought toward yourself or your healing process, force yourself to STOP it immediately. This will take practice since we are in such a habit of having negative thoughts.

   Let's say you just thought, "I will never get better." Instead, tell yourself, "I am doing everything in my power to heal." Notice your words remain true, pro-active, and positive—not demanding. You don't want to say: "I will get better." Your healing is a process and you are actively participating, and your affirmations to yourself should reflect that.

3. **Have Fun!**

    As much as possible (every day if you can!), do something that's going to make you laugh. Practice silly walks in your living room, or make funny faces at your cat or dog. Watch a funny movie or a YouTube video. Do something totally weird and spontaneous!

4. **Be Kind**

    Every week, do something nice for another person. Call or send flowers to a friend who's having a hard time. Buy a stranger a cup of coffee, give a homeless person $10, smile at the barista when she's really busy. I sometimes buy my grocery clerk a piece of chocolate, or cookie. It'll make you feel good. And remember, that energy is like a boomerang, so it does come back to you. Put out good energy whenever you can.

3rd Fundamental
Navigate Fear

MOLLY

Molly was terrified; that much was obvious. She sat down in my office and said, "I know my blood pressure is going to be way high ..." She let the statement trail off, as if her knowing might somehow take away the problem. She was nervous, pale, and she was right—her heart was literally racing.

It turned out I was the source of her fear: she was terrified of doctors.

Molly had been referred to me by a friend who had explained that my approach to medicine was "unconventional." She hoped I might be able to help Molly find ease.

Molly told me she had lost both of her parents a few years ago, one to cancer and the other to heart failure. For her, the experience of their passing was hor-

rendous. They were both misdiagnosed, and their treatments were painful and problematic. Her father spent months in the intensive care unit, and her mother suffered greatly throughout her treatment, and their respective doctors seemed indifferent to their plight. This prolonged and painful experience left Molly deeply traumatized. She had completely lost her faith in the medical profession. She was terrified to have to see a doctor for her own issues.

Molly came to my office with lower back pain, but as we spoke, it became clear that her main concern was that she was afraid she had cancer. She had been too afraid to bring it up at first. Her fear and distrust of the medical system was so great that she could not bring herself to get the necessary tests to prove whether she had cancer or not.

I performed a series of acupuncture treatments that I've developed for post-traumatic stress disorder (PTSD) in order to help heal the trauma that she experienced when her parents were dying. With PTSD, your energy is stuck in a certain place. Often, people feel that their life has never been the same since the trauma moment. The acupuncture treatments address emotional and spiritual energies that are stuck, opening up the channels so energy can flow, and allowing the body to be more open to healing.

She was my patient for four months before she finally was able to bring herself to get tested for cancer. As it turned out, she did have cancer. But once she knew she had cancer, she faced it with amazing courage. She did chemo, radiation, surgery, and focused on taking care of her body through it all. In the end, Molly did more than survive. She healed. She bravely found the way to face her greatest fear, and in the process encountered her own strength, a strength that she hadn't known existed. For Molly, the process of healing was beyond overcoming cancer and death. For Molly, her healing was about finding the tools to courageously live!

Navigating Fear

Fear can be debilitating because it is so overwhelming. Like a tidal wave, fear washes over our rational thoughts and leaves us breathing hard, disoriented, and unable to think clearly in its wake. Ultimately, fear is the primary obstacle that gets in the way of our capacity to love because when we are fearful, it is difficult to feel love. This, however, does not mean that your love is gone; you just have to find it.

When you are afraid, there is not much room for anything else in your mind and body because the physical response to fear takes so much energy. It is difficult to know how to take care of yourself, how to listen to your body, how to trust your instincts, and how to know what is right for *you*. Fear and uncertainty intensify physical symptoms. Sometimes, the fear can even be worse than the actual physical experience of pain.

Chemically, fear is triggered when your brain *perceives* that you are in danger (the threat doesn't even have to be real!). Any sense of a peril sets off a fight, flight, or freeze response in our bodies: a racing heart, fast breathing, and tense muscles. These reactions are the result of cortisol and adrenaline (called norepinephrine in the brain) immediately pumping through your brain and body whenever you experience a threat. It causes your blood pressure to rise and your heart rate to increase. These reactions are useful because when more blood is being pumped into your brain and muscles, you are ready to think fast and run hard in a crisis situation.

The fear response is largely an *involuntary* response. It is part of your autonomic nervous system, which operates below the usual state of waking consciousness. Fear affects the same part of your nervous system that controls your heart rate, breathing, perspiration, salivation, and so on. We generally cannot consciously initiate a fear response, and when it does happen, we are basically at its mercy until it runs its course. Imagine that moment when you have had a near car accident? It takes some time for your breathing and heart rate to regulate back to normal.

1st Key: Love—Your Healing Superpower

The trick to navigating fear is in bringing our logical awareness to our experience of fear so that we can begin to create more space *within our fear response.* By its nature, fear causes us to contract, pull away, run, freeze, or fight. Very often, we feel consumed by the experience. When we approach what we fear with curiosity and awareness, we create a little distance from our fear. From that vantage point, we can see more possibilities and have a greater chance to find answers and resolution. Love, on the other hand, is expansive, generous, curious. When we put more love and awareness into those moments when we experience fear, we create more space within our experience, and therefore see more possibility and have a greater chance to find answers.

If your symptoms are causing you fear, rather than letting the fear take control, look at *why* you are feeling afraid. Do you need to get tested? Do you need to change something about how you are taking care of your body? Ironically, when it comes to fear, our rational mind helps create the gap for love to come in.

There is a delicate balance in learning how to differentiate anxiety and worry—which heightens symptoms and causes more distress unnecessarily—from a true alarm signal inside of your body. My patient Molly had what seemed like an irrational fear of cancer. She couldn't have known that she had cancer, yet the alarm inside of her was so great she couldn't ignore it. The point is to not disregard your fear altogether, but to learn to not let it rule you. Experiencing fear at different moments is inevitable, and sometimes it can even be crucial to your health and well-being.

Actions and Exercises for the 3rd Fundamental Navigate Fear and Remove Blocks

1. **Breathe**

    Most of the time when we are afraid, there is not an actual threat. Instead, we're anticipating something in the future or reliving something in the past. If you feel afraid, the first thing to do is to breathe. Become aware of being in the present—the right here, right now.

    Breathing relaxes your body and helps you calm you down: it literally sends a message to the brain to calm down! It increases the oxygen supply to your brain and resets the parasympathetic nervous system, which promotes relaxation. It also slows the heartbeat and stabilizes blood pressure, "resetting" the fight-or-flight response.

    - Whenever you experience fear, immediately take five deep breaths. Breathe in for five seconds, hold for four or five seconds, and breathe out for five seconds. Make sure that you breathe into your diaphragm. Shallow, upper respiratory breath is connected to the fight-or-flight response, so in order to receive the benefits of breathing, you want to breathe into your belly.
    - Make a daily practice of deep breathing. You can connect it to a yoga, meditation, or Tai Chi practice, or you could even do it while you're driving to work in the morning. Breathe through your nose and into your belly for even just two to three minutes a day is good. See what happens!

2. **Check the Facts**

    When you experience a new or frightening physical symptom in your body, rather than immediately jumping to alarming conclusions, ask yourself some questions. I call this *checking the facts*.

These are some of the questions I ask my patients about their symptoms:

- Focus on the sensation you are having: what does it feel like? When you relax your body and listen, is it getting worse or better?
- Always watch how long and how often this symptom occurs. If it's just a brief episode and then goes away, it's probably not dangerous. If it keeps happening, notice when and how does it start.
- If you've had this same symptom before, and you're still here, notice that. Pay attention and see if the symptom is different now. If not, then whatever is going on, you know you've survived it. Take some deep breaths and see if you can get more information about it from your body.
- Is everything functioning properly? For example, if it's abdominal pain, are you still digesting food? Are you able to eat?
- What makes it better? What makes it worse? What was happening when it started?

These questions can usually guide you on how to proceed. If this is really a crisis, call 911 or get urgent help. I have included a list of emergency symptoms in Appendix B for your reference.

If it feels like you need to see a doctor, make an appointment. If you know your ailment is not life-threatening, perhaps you still need a medical test to diagnose the problem.

If there is something to be afraid of, what can you do about it? Gather together the people and means that will help you handle that issue. Take logical action that will help take care of your fear. Get support. Get help.

3. **Single Focus**

    When you experience a new and frightening symptom or feeling and start to feel overwhelmed or anxious, you can shift the anxiety by focusing on one sensation at a time. Start by breathing deeply and relaxing your body as much as possible, then pay attention to ONE sensation. Let's say you're feeling pain in your chest, your heart is beating fast, and it's hard to get a deep breath. Start by focusing on the pain; just breathe and notice the pain. Don't let the other symptoms distract you, just keep focusing on the pain. It usually takes a minute or two for the sensation to shift.

    Then you can move on and pay attention to another sensation. Usually when we are frightened, we are also overwhelmed with too many sensations. So, by focusing on one sensation at a time, we are able to "reduce the noise," which will help calm us down.

4th Fundamental
The Essence of Balance—Everything Is Connected

THE DANCE OF YIN AND YANG

In Chinese philosophy, which is deeply rooted in Taoism, the two principles that create balance in the universe are Yin and Yang—the harmony of opposites. Yin and Yang exist within each of us, and in everything. Down to the tiniest cell, every element of energy has a Yin component and a Yang component.

Most people are familiar with the symbol of Yin and Yang—the black and white circle that perfectly illustrates their interaction. Each side of the circle contains the seed of the other. One side is not superior and the circle cannot be complete without the other. Just as night needs day, Yin and Yang create a totality, a complete whole. They rely upon each other to exist, and their relationship is dynamic, completely interdependent, and constantly seeking balance.

The principles of Yin and Yang—of balance and harmony—underlie everything in Chinese medicine. They will come up again and again later in this book, but for now, we are examining the *relationship* between Yin and Yang.

Yin (the black of the circle) is the passive principle of the universe, characterized as feminine and sustaining. It is associated with the earth, and energetically, Yin is dark, moist, soft, cold, nighttime, moonlight, underneath, and emotional.

Yang (the white of the circle) is the active principle of the universe, characterized as masculine and creative. It is associated with heaven, and energetically, Yang is sunny, bright, hot, dry, hard, daytime, and on top.

The symbol of Yin and Yang is circular because it never ends—the movement toward equilibrium is happening all the time. Like the push and pull of the waves of the ocean, or like our breath, Yin and Yang are constantly moving in and out, giving and receiving. They are like lovers in an epic romance, dancing individually and yet as one, and their relationship is one of constantly seeking balance and a shared sense of wholeness.

We all dance with the changing energies in our lives. Our careers and families, our thoughts and feelings, where we live, and even the weather play a part in this dance. Through life's ups and downs, we naturally and intuitively shift with the tides, always seeking that place of balance where life is flowing smoothly.

As we all know, life is not always smooth. A physical trauma, a bad fight with a loved one, prolonged lack of movement, a poor diet, toxins in the environment, or chronic stress can cause an imbalance in your body. Sometimes an emotional reaction can trigger a thought process that causes you to worry, and if you are not able to release the emotion, your energy may become stuck. When this happens, and particularly if this kind of reaction becomes an emotional pattern, your natural, inner equilibrium can go off-kilter and become stuck, or stagnant.

Usually, an imbalance of any nature—physical, emotional, mental, or spiritual—starts out as a slight irritation in the body, but if it's not addressed, it can develop into something more pronounced. In our bodies, imbalance begins on an energetic level, and then moves into the blood, and eventually into the tissue. When you are healthy and you feel good, your energy is flowing easily, smoothly, and rhythmically—just like a dance. Physical pain usually means that energy is stuck in your body.

Our immediate reaction to pain is to want to get rid of it, to take medication to dull the pain—but it is important to remember that when your body hurts, it is trying to help you address something important. You can take the pain medication, but also try to find what may be causing the imbalance or "stuckness". Chinese medicine uses acupuncture, herbs, and other modalities to help move your energy and re-establish the inherent equilibrium in your body.

Everything Is Connected

Chinese medicine describes in precise detail the relationships that exist within the body, which are all rooted in the dance of Yin and Yang. Chinese medicine explains how *everything* is connected and interrelated. Your extremities, senses, muscles, and bones are all affected by your organs and they each affect and influence one another. At the same time, your emotions, your will, and your spirit are constantly working in relationship to each other and to your body. *Therefore, everything you do and experience is connected, and an important part of your healing.*

According to Chinese medicine, your whole body is affected when one part is out of alignment. You cannot just heal your arm when it is broken. Your body, mind, emotions, and spirit all *equally* participate in your healing. This means that when you hate your body or your experiences—like the pain of that broken arm, or the person you think is responsible for your broken arm—it affects your whole being: it affects how you heal. You want to do everything in your power to get rid of the pain, but instead of hating it, focus on the fact that *you are healing*.

Pain is one side of an experience. Yin and Yang show us that the other side exists—it *has to* exist. One side gives rise to the other, so that even in the darkest night, we know that the sun will rise again.

Love is intrinsic to the dance between Yin and Yang. Love is the energy between the two sides; science shows us that it eases friction and assists flow. Love helps you find the good. When you focus on love, even when you are in pain, it changes your whole experience. As the Hero of your journey, imagine that compassion and love are your magic tools. Love will help you find balance and open the door to greater healing.

Actions and Exercises for the 4th Fundamental
The Essence of Balance

1. **Create a Garden Inside of You**
   Anytime you feel your thoughts or your emotions becoming negative, which can spiral into feelings of hopelessness, put all of your effort into creating a "garden" inside of yourself. And just like tending a garden, this requires consistent attentiveness, because our negative thoughts can take root and convince us that we're never going to feel better. Instead, you can visualize yourself turning away from those ugly thoughts and begin to create an amazing, magical garden inside your heart and mind. In this garden, love flows in the rivers and the sunlight. Imagine your favorite flowers. Imagine fruit trees, and the sunlight coming through and reflecting off the dew on the leaves. Imagine an abundance of beauty and light

and sweet scents inside of you. Get creative. Engage all your senses in this oasis!

Each time dark thoughts arise, remember this beautiful garden that exists inside of you. Its beauty is powerful: it can absorb the darkness in its light. As Anne Frank said, *"Look how a single candle can both defy and define the darkness."*

2. **Distraction**

Sometimes when you're in pain, all you can seem to think about is the pain. One tried and true method for pain relief is distraction, or focusing your energy on something else. Cook a meal, knit a sweater, take a walk, spend time with a loved one, watch a movie, listen to your favorite music, or turn your attention to a project you're wanting to get done. If you're busy with something else, you won't be focusing on your pain.

3. **Tree Pose**

The tree pose in Yoga is all about balance. If you're unfamiliar with yoga, you can simply try balancing your weight on one foot. Lean against a wall to begin if you feel unsteady (you don't want to fall down!). By focusing on balancing your body, you actually increase your focus and balance in your whole being.

4. **Dance with Your Own Energy**

Many years ago when I studied Aikido, we would begin our practice by allowing our bodies to move with the energy we were holding. It is a great way to release any emotional energy we have. The practice is called *Katsugen Undo* in the Aikido tradition. Begin to create a gentle movement with your breath to release stuck energy. Remember, pain is caused by stuck energy, so releasing it will help.

Begin by breathing deeply. As you breathe out, bundle yourself in a ball, contracting your body and allowing yourself to feel whatever is coming out. Then, as you breathe in, expand your body, stretch your arms out, expand in every way. Expand and contract with your breath; breathe in and breathe out. Feel the dance that is happening in your body, and if you want, begin to move your body more. Keep breathing with your movements. As the energy dissipates, you will slowly come to a stop when it is done.

If this feels good to you, try doing this every day for 30 days. See what happens!

5th Fundamental
Community Support

THE "CURE" FOR LONELINESS

One of the hardest things about being sick is that it can be terribly lonely. You are the only one who can be inside your body and fully know what you are experiencing. We crave connection, but when we are sick, we also tend to isolate. Feeling vulnerable and weak, it sometimes just feels safer to be alone since we have more control over our environment.

Although isolating may sometimes *feel* like the right thing to do, if taken to an extreme it can make you even more unwell. Studies have shown that people who are socially isolated release more cortisol, which causes inflammation and weakens the immune system. Loneliness can affect everything from hormones, to heart health, to our ability to heal. Physical diseases that are caused or exacerbated by loneliness include: Alzheimer's, obesity, diabetes, high blood pressure, heart disease, neurodegenerative diseases, and even cancer. Tumors can metastasize faster in lonely people. Extreme loneliness has been shown to be equivalent to smoking as a health risk!

It's important to note that loneliness is not just about being physically alone. It has more to do with feeling cared for and connected to others.

These days, it seems that loneliness is becoming an epidemic. Even though the world has become "smaller," people feel that they are relating less and less in authentic or "real" ways. A recent study by Cigna Health surveyed 20,000 Americans and found that 47% of them experience loneliness or the feeling of being left out. (Polack 5/2018)

So, what can we do about this epidemic of loneliness, which just seems to keep growing? And when we are ill, or feel wretched and in pain, how can we avoid the trap of isolating ourselves and being consumed by our sense of loneliness?

VULNERABILITY

Dr. Brené Brown gives a wonderful TED Talk where she explains that expressing our vulnerability is what allows us to connect more deeply with others. She describes that feelings of belonging, love, joy, courage, and creativity ultimately stem from our vulnerability.

Her research shows that people who are afraid of connection, or feel they are not worthy of love, tend to separate themselves from others. According to Dr. Brown's research, in order to truly feel connected to others, we first have to feel *worthy* of belonging and love. She has shown that people have deeper connections with others when they see vulnerability as a strength, and as something that is important and natural. Those people *have a desire to express themselves*, even when they are in pain.

On some level, our very survival feels threatened when we are sick because illness affects our ability to function in the world. Yet, as a species, our survival has always been tied to our ability to support each other and work together. We cannot do it all alone, and we were never meant to.

Possibly one of the greatest gifts of being sick is that it puts you in a position to receive help. Powerhouse people have to let go of their extreme self-reliance and depend upon others when they are sick. Illness allows you to be a recipient of care. It is a chance for people to come together and support you.

Perhaps when we isolate—not wanting to trouble other people with our pain—we are actually depriving our loved ones of an opportunity to be connecting, loving, and caring for us. Finding ways to be vulnerable when we are sick is healthy for everyone involved. I have seen illness, and the process of healing, open the hearts of my patients and their loved ones again and again.

BUILDING COMMUNITY

Science has proven that feeling connected to others strengthens our longevity, gives meaning to our lives, builds community, and is ultimately essential to our survival. Illness can become a catalyst toward creating deeper connection, compassion, and understanding by learning to express how we are feeling when we are sick and being willing to receive help from others. Research at the Institute of HeartMath shows that when people are in some sort of trouble in their lives, or in their bodies, or in need of some other sort of help, heart energy actually extends out from their bodies, apparently looking for connection.

Sometimes there is not a community to support an individual. Sometimes, due to circumstances—living in remote areas, or just the fast-paced scale of life itself—it feels like there is no one to help out. I've worked with many people who feel terribly alone in their illness. If you are struggling with feeling isolated and alone, there are things you can do to feel more connected. You can participate in support groups, either physically or online. If you have the energy, you can volunteer with an organization that you feel passionate about.

According to a 2007 study by the National Corp. for Community Service, (Grimm, Spring, Dietz, 2007) volunteering improves health, mortality, and well-being. It also lessens symptoms of chronic pain and heart disease—even more than paid work—especially with volunteers 65 years and older.

You can get a dog, a cat, or maybe a goldfish. Even a plant that you can care for can help. When something requires nurturing, it will also nurture you.

I know that taking the initiative to connect with others when you are sick can be super challenging. For some people, it may seem impossible. Start with something small, a call to an old friend or family member. Care sometimes comes from unexpected places. Don't be afraid to tell them what you're experiencing. Remember, it is a great feat and takes great courage to be vulnerable. As the *Tao Te Ching* states, "By compassion, one can be brave." Always remember that finding the willingness and the ability to express what is in your heart is an act of great courage.

Actions and Exercises for the 5th Fundamental Community Support

1. **Talk to people about your experiences.** Be willing to be vulnerable and share what you've felt and learned. Even if it's just with one person, find someone you can trust. When you share your experiences, you naturally begin to observe and gain more understanding for what is happening, and it can be greatly illuminating for both you and your friends and supporters.

2. **Invite others to share their experiences with you.** Part of the magic of being vulnerable is that you give others permission to be vulnerable as well. Sometimes, when someone is going through something very painful, the listener may feel that they should not talk about themselves. But when the listener shares their own experiences, more *relating* can happen. It also helps take your mind off of what you are going through,

and creates a deeper line of connection between you.

3. **Find healers who support you.** You should feel comfortable and have open lines of communication with your healers. Every relationship is unique and has its ups and downs, so every time you see your doctor or healer, it may not be perfect. The important thing is to feel that you can openly share what you are experiencing, and that they understand and can help you feel better.

4. **Find people who will support you.** Help sometimes arrives in unlikely packages, so be open to some out-of-the-box friendships and support. There are so many online support groups and opportunities to interact— through Facebook communities, online forums, or meet-up groups on healing. There might be support groups at your local hospital.

    Maybe your community is not one cohesive group of people, but instead many people from different parts of your life. This is your healing family; let them in.

5. **Hug a tree.** There are now many studies that show that interacting with trees and plants can help with depression, concentration, and self-discipline, and can even reduce headaches.

    Find a tree near your home that you can go to easily, every day if possible. Hug the tree with your chest against it, or sit or squat with your body touching the tree, or just put your hands it. Feel the energy of the tree as it radiates into you. You might actually feel that the tree hugs you back!

6. **Rediscover a passion from your childhood.** If you always liked art, take an art class. Do something unexpected. Shake up your world and see

what happens. You might find new soulmates by doing the things you love to do.

7. **Exercise.** According to the Cigna study, people who exercise are considerably less lonely than those who don't. Join an exercise class, which will increase your chance of finding other people to connect with. Many of my patients have formed social connections with classmates in their yoga studio or dance classes.

Chapter 2

2nd Key: Physical Balance and Vitality

"To Western Medicine, understanding an illness means uncovering a distinct entity that is separate from the patient's being; to Chinese Medicine, understanding means perceiving the relationships between all the patient's signs and symptoms in the context of his or her life."
—TED KAPTCHUK, THE WEB THAT HAS NO WEAVER

JOYCE

The first time I spoke with Joyce she was in tears. She had been suffering relentless nausea and intense stomach pain for three solid months. Unable to eat, she had lost 20 pounds from her already thin frame. She was desperate.

Joyce had seen expert physicians from UCSF and Stanford and had taken every conceivable test, but all test results came back negative. No one could figure out what was wrong with her. She had tried medications for nausea, acid blockers, motility medications (designed to help the stomach move and digest food), and even antidepressants, but she had found no relief.

At 60 years old, Joyce had experienced mild anxiety for most of her life. Her normal response was a loss of appetite, but the symptoms were never this bad. When she first contacted me to see if I might help her, I told her I'd seen this problem many times, and that I could definitely help.

According to my knowledge of Chinese medicine, I felt confident we would *find that Joyce had an imbalance in her spleen.*

The spleen produces blood, which is the primary function according to our Western medical understanding. According to Chinese medicine, it is also responsible for a person's ability to take in food, transform that food into energy, and transport the energy throughout the body. It regulates the strength of muscles, the ability to concentrate, and the emotions of worry and anxiety.

All of Joyce's symptoms corresponded to a spleen imbalance, but in Western medicine, there are no tests available that could diagnose her problem. I used Chinese medicine to treat her ailment. I gave her herbs and specific acupuncture treatments for her spleen, and prescribed a diet of only cooked foods, eaten at certain times, which helped make it easier for her spleen to heal so her body could absorb the food.

Within one week of my treatments to her, Joyce was able to eat food again without pain. It took another three weeks for her to begin gaining weight, but she quickly began to feel hopeful rather than anxious about her health and well-being, which greatly improved her healing process.

ABC's

During my ten years as an ER physician, there was a specific protocol we followed when a person came into the ER with trauma. This was to ensure that we didn't miss anything—that nothing beyond the obvious was wrong. Someone who was hit by a car might have many problems, not just an obvious fractured leg. So we would wait for the patient to arrive, and then start with the *"ABC's."* First, we would make sure the *Airway* was functioning. Then, we would assess that the patient was *Breathing*. Finally, we would check their *Circulation*, looking for places that the patient was losing blood, or where circulation was impaired. Often, in the case of trauma, a person might have internal bleeding, which we wouldn't be able to see without looking for it.

After finishing the ABC's, we would then examine the body from head to toe using X-rays and visual exams. The life of each patient depended upon

2nd Key: Physical Balance and Vitality

our tenacity, thoroughness, and ability to pay attention to more than just the obvious symptoms. In the ER, missing one thing could be a matter of life or death.

When I went into private practice, I kept that mindset. I approached each patient with the intention of finding all the possible physical things that could be wrong, rather than just listening to the chief complaint. Chinese medicine naturally supports this very thorough philosophy of exam, diagnosis, and treatment, but it takes diagnosis a step further. It works to locate the root of the problem: the overall imbalance and the source of the symptoms.

The majority of my work is about creating balance in the body as a whole. Rather than taking a problem at face value, I find a way to bring your body into greater balance—not quite ignoring the symptoms that drove you to seek help, but looking beyond them to find the root cause. That way your body can heal, no matter what. Even if I don't know exactly why a particular problem is happening, I can support and balance the whole body, which in turn alleviates the specific symptoms—as in the case of Ellen.

UNDERSTANDING THE 2ND KEY

If you are ill or injured, the 2nd Key addresses the *physical aspect* of your issue. The tumor, torn ligament, broken bone, cancer, fever, phlegmy cough, rash—these symptoms usually need to be addressed through some sort of physical care. Even conditions that don't appear to be physical, including depression, anxiety, or issues that cannot be diagnosed through conventional tests, have physical components that need to be relieved for healing to occur.

The 2nd Key is about seeking and gaining support through various types of medical treatment which generally involves support from an external source. When you have someone listen to your lungs, or you have an X-ray, or receive other diagnostic tests and evaluations, these are specific actions that focus on altering your physical state. The resulting medical prescriptions, including surgery (if it's indicated) and other modalities like acupuncture, chiropractic, massage, herbs, and homeopathy, all make up the 2nd Key. These treatments should ultimately help *begin* to bring your body back to balance.

The 2nd Key is what helps you move you out of a crisis state, so that you can begin to address the other Keys and truly heal.

ONE OF SEVEN

You might think that addressing the physical is the *definition* of medicine, but as we delve into the 7 Keys, we learn that the physical is just the *one* of *seven* vital healing elements. This is arguably the most significant and most revolutionary element of the 2nd Key: it is only *one* of *seven*. Our health is dependent upon integrating all aspects of our being in order to achieve wholeness.

Western medicine is slowly moving toward a more holistic healing model of medicine. The development of neuroscience and hormone technologies is ramping up, and the effect of the emotions on health is becoming more empirical. Science is finally proving what Chinese medicine has practiced for so long.

The merging—or at least intersection—of Western and Chinese medicine offers us the best of all worlds in medicine. As a health provider, it is very exciting to be on the leading edge of the changing health paradigm, and to be able to offer my blended approach to my patients, which has yielded such tremendous results.

Fundamentals of the 2nd Key
Physical Balance and Vitality

When you are sick or injured, caring for the physical factors of your health restores a sense of wholeness and balance and allows room for the other six keys to work.

In the case of a severe illness like cancer, you may have periods of time when you are engaged in chemotherapy, radiation, or surgical treatment, and the treatment takes 100% of your energy. These treatments are very much reflections of the 2nd Key. At the same time, part of the power of the 2nd Key is in learning to attend to the whole of you, and not just the problem areas. When your whole body is in balance, it is easier to heal.

Below are the fundamental elements that frame the 2nd Key:

1st Fundamental: The Triangle of Wellness

The first fundamental of the 2nd Key takes your focus away from your symptoms, or from the Western diagnosis that you have received, so that you can begin to see yourself as a whole. The *Triangle of Wellness* is a healing principle I've developed that is based on my unique blend of Chinese and Western medicine. The *Triangle* is made up of three points: the hormones, the immune system, and the nervous system. These three systems affect every aspect of your health. When these systems are balanced, your body can begin to heal, no matter your current physical condition.

2nd Fundamental: Finding the Root Cause
Part of healing is figuring out what caused your body to go out of balance in the first place. If you can get to the source of the issue, you have a much better chance of healing, rather than simply managing the symptoms. In locating and addressing the root of imbalance, you won't end up in the same place of imbalance in six months—or even five years—down the line. Working with an expert is usually the most expedient method to uncover the root of a physical issue. This is usually done with your doctor or healer through physical exams, taking tests, studying labs, and in-depth inquiry.

3rd Fundamental: Cultivating Curiosity and Exploring Healing Methods
Approaching your health with curiosity allows you to find what is best for you. Any time you feel angry or hopeless, invite yourself to become curious. Asking questions that begin with, "I wonder…?" opens you up to possibility, and within possibility lives hope. Becoming curious might initiate exploration into healing modalities that can restore your body's balance, including hormone balancing, supplements, herbs, acupuncture, surgery (as indicated), prescriptions, breath work, stress reduction techniques, physical therapy, and other hands-on healing techniques. Be determined to find the method, or methods, that work best *for you.*

4th Fundamental: Building Your Relationship with Your Healthcare Provider and Healing Team
Trust is a crucial element to healing. Find the right people to help you with your journey of healing. You may need more than one practitioner, but each one should be someone you feel good about. By creating a positive relationship with the experts who are helping you heal, you are building the foundation for a vibrant, healthy life.

2nd Key: Physical Balance and Vitality

1st Fundamental
The Triangle of Wellness

"Balancing your hormones, immune system, and nervous system creates the structure for healing to occur."
—SHIROKO SOKITCH, MD

MIKE

Mike had fibromyalgia—a chronic pain in his muscles. Mike was 60 when he first came to see me and had been suffering chronic upper back and arm pain for more than six years. The pain was relentless. He was living on painkillers every day just to be able to function. He had seen countless doctors, but no one had an answer for him. His long history of sleeping poorly, his bad diet, and his low sex drive had never been addressed.

On his first visit, he also told me that he had been having marital difficulties for years. He felt he couldn't communicate well with his wife, and that she didn't understand how he was feeling physically.

Mike had classical imbalances of the "Triangle of Wellness." His hormones, nervous system, immune system and digestion were all functioning poorly. We started by changing his diet and weaning him off the medications that were destroying his digestion. Then we began balancing his hormones using bio-identical hormone replacement therapy, acupuncture, and nutritional supplements. It took about six months to get him to feel more balanced. All the actions we took allowed him to build his energy and have the substrate for healing.

Once he felt more nourished and was receiving hormonal and immune support, he began to feel better and have less pain. As he felt better, he also began to have fun and enjoy his wife again, healing their marriage.

Hormones, Immune System, and Nervous System

When you have pain in one part of your body, remember that even while you are trying to resolve that pain, it is affecting the rest of your body. Your hormones can go more and more out of balance due to the stress of the pain and the energy required to sustain your body when it's hurting. If you take painkillers, you can have digestive problems and even liver imbalance from the medication. Stress and digestive issues will also affect your brain chemistry and weaken your immune system.

The important thing to remember about the 2nd Key of physical balance is that when you are in pain, you want to find ways to support your whole body, rather than just focusing on the part causing you pain. This is where the *Triangle of Wellness* comes into play. These three systems—hormones, nervous system, immune system—are deeply interdependent. If any one of them is functioning poorly it will affect the other three, and their proper function and balance supports every other element of our health. Balancing the *Triangle of Wellness* facilitates the treatment and healing of your medical condition, no matter your condition.

When you have been ill for a long time, or have a serious chronic medical condition, the *Triangle of Wellness* is usually out of balance. Unfortunately, if it's not addressed, it will be affected more and more over time. If you are experiencing a chronic health problem, you should consider having these systems reviewed and tested. You can talk to your doctor about what would be the best tests for you to take (and I have also listed some tests that I recommend in Appendix B at the end of the book).

Hormones

Hormones affect the body in myriad ways, but they remain fairly mysterious to most people. We think of them when they are more amplified during certain times, like in puberty, pregnancy, or menopause, but these are just the sex hormones!

2nd Key: Physical Balance and Vitality

Hormones are the body's chemical messengers. There are seven hormone-producing glands in your body and each regulates a variety of functions, including: digestion, blood sugar, metabolism, bone and muscle strength, sleep, stress response, focus, energy levels, sexual function, growth and development, reproduction, and mood.

If your hormones are balanced and functioning as they are intended, every aspect of your physical and emotional health is positively affected. On the other hand, if your hormones are out of balance for any other reason, your whole body will be negatively affected.

Hormones do not operate in isolation, but in concert with other hormones. Their proper function is assisted by the brain. When I review a person's hormone results, I explain to them that it is not so much the individual numbers that matter, but that one hormone relies upon another for support.

For example, if your cortisol (the stress hormone) is particularly high or low, it may or may not affect your energy right away, since other hormones may be picking up the slack. The problem is, if there is an imbalance, eventually you will be affected. Your hormones work together in a great balancing act; their proper functioning is determined by their relationship to one another.

The reasons our hormones go out of balance are numerous. The biggest factors that affect our hormones are stress (most people live with their stress response turned "on" all the time), poor diet (especially a diet high in sugar, salt, and processed carbohydrates), specific food allergies, toxins, chemicals, heavy metals, fake hormones in the environment (pesticides used on vegetables, hormones fed to beef, pork, and chicken, and plastics), chronic illness, infections, and changes in life patterns.

If your body is not behaving how you think it should, it's likely your hormones have something to do with it. Proper rest, exercise, and eating healthy are three very immediate things that you can do to help begin to balance your hormones and reduce stress. In addition, once you have your hormones tested, there are supplements and herbs that work wonders at helping to create balance in the body.

Nervous System

The nervous system remains one of the most complex and mysterious systems in modern science. It is the "computer" in your body that runs the whole show, yet our knowledge and understanding of it has only just begun! We have learned more about the vital and intricate processes of the nervous system in the past 20 years than we did in the millennia before, and what we know is still just the tip of the iceberg!

The nervous system includes your brain, spinal cord, and all of the nerves in your body. Your brain and nerves communicate with every part of your body, constantly sending signals that are channeled back and forth throughout your body via neurotransmitters. Your brain sends the signals that your hormones receive, so your brain is actually in charge of your hormones!

Every single thing that happens to you all day long is recorded in your nervous system. Everything you touch and feel, your thoughts, your heartbeat, your ability to digest food, and your breathing are just a few important examples of what is connected to your nervous system. It is always on the alert for signals that are dangerous. When you make a move, it is your nervous system telling you to make a move. Basically, everything that you experience, *and* your body's proper functioning, is run by your nervous system.

Scientists used to think that if your brain was damaged, it couldn't heal. It was thought that any function a person regained after a neurologic trauma was because of a new learning, or calling a different part of the nervous system into play. We now know that every element of your brain and nervous system can heal—especially if we nourish the brain correctly. We nourish the brain with our thoughts, our diet, our behaviors, with exercise, and by healing our digestive system.

Recent science reveals that your guts have an entire, complicated nervous

2nd Key: Physical Balance and Vitality

system of their own. There are neurological (nervous system) processes that happen in the lining of the intestines that never make it to the brain. So it's not just your brain that rules your nervous system—your gut has key neurological connections, too.

One example of a gut neurological process is the production of serotonin. Serotonin is a neurotransmitter that is associated with feelings of happiness and well-being, and scientific studies have determined that you make more serotonin in your gut than in your brain. With this knowledge, we can understand that our diet and digestion deeply affects not only how we feel physically, but also our emotional well-being.

IMMUNE SYSTEM

Each day, all day long, you have bacteria and viruses on your skin and inside your body that *could* cause an infection. Why do you *not* get sick? And why does your body sometimes let down its defenses?

According to Chinese medicine, there are two ways that people become sick: through internal and external influences. External influences come from outside the body: infectious diseases, environmental causes, and allergens. Internal influences are rooted in the emotions. We will address how our health is affected by our emotions in greater detail in Chapter 5. For now, we can understand that when you feel overly stressed, worried, depressed, helpless, or angry, these emotions can actually deplete your immune system and make you more susceptible to illness.

Chinese Medicine describes the energy of your body as working in layers. Simply put, the outermost organ of your body is the skin, which is regulated by your lungs. The innermost organ is your bones, regulated by the kidneys. In the middle is the blood, which is regulated by the liver.

The lungs and large intestines are both associated with the outermost layer of your body's energy. They act as barriers to the outside world, and are connected to the immune system. They defend your body from foreign invaders, including bacteria, parasites, and viruses.

The outer layers of energy are most susceptible to outside influences. If an illness that begins in the outer layers is treated properly, it will not necessarily progress into the inner layers of energy.

Ninety percent of the time that you become sick, it starts in the outermost layer—the lungs, the nose, the throat, or the large intestines (diarrhea). A cold or flu invades the body through the lungs or large intestine, and if it isn't treated properly, it can cause long-term illness. The kidneys, which reside in the innermost layer of your body's energy, are generally only affected once an illness has progressed.

Your immune system is your internal defense mechanism, your ability to protect yourself from outside world. It helps you remain healthy. The tissues that are a part of the immune system itself include white blood cells, the lymphatic system, and the spleen. Like a sentinel in a camp, your immune system is tuned to recognize what doesn't belong, deny its entrance, and kick it out. It is constantly battling the viruses and microbes in your body, and constantly protecting you from what might harm you.

If your immune system is strong, it means that you heal quickly, you don't often become sick, your digestion is working well, and you have few or no allergies. Part of building a strong immune system is actually getting sick. This is why children get sick so much more than adults: their bodies are learning how to protect, adapt, and heal illnesses.

What makes the difference between a strong or weak immune system? Why does that strep bacteria sit in your throat most days without any difficulty and then suddenly it's an infection? These things occur because our energy goes out of balance. It could be an emotional trigger, such as feeling overwhelmed by how much you have to do, or having to deal with your family during the holidays. Or, you might be overworked and exhausted and not getting enough rest. Or, your body is already challenged with some other issue, making it difficult to fight two things at the same time. Or, you may need to express yourself more to be in balance mentally and spiritually, and having strep is a way to put the focus on your throat.

A weak immune system can cause many problems. Working to strengthen your immune system, and properly address illnesses at the onset, are the mainstays of good health. If your immune system is overactive, that is still an imbalance of your immunity—they are both spectrums of the same problem. When your system reacts to *everything*, it means that it is upset about something, and you need to find the root cause of it.

ORGANIC GARDENING

You can think of your body as a garden. The flowering plants and vegetables of your garden are the result of you caring for your health. It is possible to put *pesticides* (*i.e.,* poor diet, processed foods, stress, lack of proper rest) in your garden. The plants will grow—they will be forced to grow. But in the end, those "chemicals" will destroy the soil, and if the soil is poor or if you fail to nurture it, you will not grow healthy plants.

Taking care of the Triangle of Wellness is like taking care of the soil in your garden. No matter what illness you may have, if these three things are balanced, you will feel better. Even when you don't know what is wrong with you, if you heal your immune system, your nervous system, and your hormones—which can take place through diet, exercise, herbs, and supplements—you have a good chance to heal anyway.

And remember: the symptom may not actually be the root of the problem. Everything is connected. This is so important! Do you remember the song, "The hip bone's connected to the thigh bone, the thigh bone's connected to the leg bone …"? Well, there are even deeper connections that science and Chinese medicine have now proven, such as your gut health being connected to your brain health, or how your outer ankle pain might reflect an issue in your gallbladder, or vice versa, or your large intestine infection might show up as a rash on your skin and *no* digestive symptoms!

The 2nd Fundamental will guide you how to dig deeper into finding the true root of your symptoms.

Actions and Exercises for the 1st Fundamental
The Triangle of Wellness

1. **Healthy living.** There are often very simple, natural things you can do to bring your hormones and nervous system into a state of greater calm and balance, which will affect how you feel on every level.

   Here are just a few ideas:
   - Practice good sleep hygiene: make sure you get to bed consistently on time, turn out the lights, put away devices, make sure your bed is comfortable for you.
   - Eat a good protein breakfast within one hour of getting up in the morning.
   - Practice deep breathing for a few minutes a day, to calm and balance your nervous system.
   - Get outside for a few minutes a day: sun and nature help balance your body.
   - Eat your vegetables! They have all sorts of healing properties.

2. **Get tested.** If you suspect that your Triangle of Wellness is out of balance, get tested by partnering with a medical or healing expert. There are many normal lab tests that can be done to assess your health status, which are covered by insurance. In addition, you can do tests that will reveal more about the deeper functions of your body systems—they are called "functional medicine tests." Some examples are the following: Adrenal hormone profile (either blood, urine or saliva—I prefer dried urine

because it reveals how your body uses hormones, not just what the levels are); specific stool tests that can reveal hidden infections looking for the DNA of potential pathogens rather than living organisms, and more. I have also listed a number of additional tests in *Appendix B* at the back of the book.

2nd Fundamental
Finding the Root Cause

CAROL

Carol was referred to me by her sister and had what seemed like an endless list of medical problems—autoimmune disease, rheumatoid arthritis, and back pain—to name a few. She was 60 years old, and she wasn't getting better. When I felt her pulse, I knew that Carol had a liver imbalance.

One of the chief methods of diagnosis in Chinese medicine is reading the pulse. This allows the practitioner to assess the state of the internal organs and energy of the body. Pulse diagnosis in Chinese medicine is complex and requires a high level of expertise. It is very different than the standard heart rate pulse that is measured in Western medicine.

I treated Carol with acupuncture to alleviate her pain, and I told her about the liver imbalance. Unfortunately, she never came back to see me, due to financial and insurance issues. But I did receive a call from her sister a month later. She told me that Carol had been diagnosed with liver cancer.

With Chinese medicine diagnostic tools, I could not have known definitively that Carol had cancer, but my diagnosis propelled her to ask her doctor for the tests she needed. One of the things I love about Chinese Medicine is that I am able to see the patient through different eyes, which can then guide my use of Western medicine.

Getting to the Root of the Problem

Any chronic or unresolved symptom deeply affects how we relate to the world, what we are able to achieve, and how we feel, both emotionally and spiritually. Often, these issues start off gently. You may not even remember the initial event. Perhaps you had a flu virus or a cold that didn't heal in the way that it should, or a mild injury that you ignored. Maybe something stressful, like a big deadline, happened at work, or maybe your boss just seems angry most the time. Maybe one of your family members was sick and you had to take care of him or her, and you lost sleep in the process. These minor events can all build into something much greater over time.

Finding the root of a problem means being able to understand your body's energy. Chinese medicine practitioners do this by feeling the pulse and looking at the tongue: it's like taking a snapshot of your energy and learning where the problem lies. Once I understand the imbalance in my patient, I can use testing in Western medicine to diagnose the root cause more deeply. Tests include anything from routine blood tests, to more in-depth evaluations including stool tests to analyze your digestion, urine hormone tests, or more advanced assessments like an organic acids test to learn how your entire metabolism is working and whether you are overloaded with toxins.

When a new patient comes into my office, I spend an hour and a half with them at that initial visit. We discuss their health, their physical issues and concerns, and what they would like to achieve. I ask a lot of questions about symptoms, past history, and lifestyle. I'm also looking for where the story began. It could even have begun at the time of conception!

2nd Key: Physical Balance and Vitality

There are four important elements to consider when you are trying to find the root of an issue:
1. *Jing*
2. Lifestyle
3. Digestion
4. Present time: What is happening in your life now and what was happening when the issue began.

Below is a description of these four factors, followed by exercises to help you dive into both your history and the current state of your life. The goal is to uncover where your current health issue originates.

JING AND GENES

Finding the root of an issue may mean going back as far as the day you were born, or even before!

Jing is your life force energy or your essence. We originally receive Jing—our innate Jing—from our parents. It is housed in the kidneys. Jing is similar to DNA or genetics, but in addition to genomes, Jing is also affected by what your parents were experiencing when they conceived you, how healthy they were at the time, and the conditions of your birth experience. Ideally, your healthy parents created you in a loving conscious environment, and spent the time they were pregnant with you taking great care of their health, and nurturing you from the earliest beginning. But that is obviously not always the case.

Genetics has always been seen as fairly fixed, yet research is now showing that lifestyle factors can change your genetic expression, even as an adult. Recent science shows we can affect our genetics by how we live: this is known as the science of "epigenetics." Our genetics can be healed—which means that no one should feel condemned to a certain life or lifestyle because of their genes. At the same time, it is helpful to look at where you've come from to help guide your decisions and learn where you might need to pay special attention.

A great book about this subject by Dr. Ben Lynch—*Dirty Genes*, published in 2018—talks about how we have certain genetic tendencies that can affect our health in many ways. He lays out a list of symptoms of various genetic imbalances, and what to do about them.

Childhood trauma is another element that affects Jing. A study on Adverse Childhood Events (ACE's) reveals that people who experience many traumatic events as children are more likely to suffer chronic illness as adults. (Felitti, Anda, et al, 1998.) This study has generated a lot of research since it was done, showing how much trauma can affect your physical health, and it is certainly a thing to keep in mind as a root cause.

Understanding your history and your innate Jing can help you understand why you might be susceptible to certain medical conditions. You may have certain predispositions, but the great thing about Jing is that you can build it or deplete it, depending upon how you live your life. The idea is that you either burn out your essence or continue to fuel yourself through healthy living. The good news is, even if you are born with low Jing, you can change the results.

LIFESTYLE HISTORY

When you have a longstanding or difficult health problem, every element of your individual story plays a role in your health. Possible examples of conditions that may cause ongoing imbalance are: infections, toxins, emotional stresses, mold in homes or workplaces, heavy metals, overexposure to certain foods—like sugar, wheat, corn, dairy, soy, or eggs—or too much or too little exercise.

There may be habits you enjoy now that are affecting your health in a negative manner. One patient, I remember, drank a 12 pack of coca-cola every day, and then wondered why he had trouble sleeping. It never occurred to him that it might affect his sleep.

You may not know that you are sensitive to a certain food, such as nightshades. My patient Kevin came to me with Rheumatoid Arthritis, and when I asked him about night shades—such as potatoes, tomatoes, eggplant and all peppers—which can cause Rheumatoid arthritis symptoms, he said that he didn't eat any of that. Then a few minutes later he said, "Wait, are potato chips and salsa night shades?" When he quit eating them, all his symptoms improved.

These are obviously extreme examples, but we all have places in our lives where we might be missing something that, to another person, may seem totally obvious. When you are searching for the root cause, don't leave anything out—leave no stone unturned.

Digestion

Digestion is your body's ability to take in, break down, and absorb nutrients. It affects every element of your overall health. If your digestion isn't working, it's hard to get the nutrition you need to heal. Digestion, like the rest of your body, requires hormones, immunity, and nervous system in order to function. More and more research is showing that digestive issues are at the root of many other chronic health conditions.

You may have ignored seemingly minor digestive issues for years, or you may not even have any digestive symptoms, but your digestion is very often the root cause of health issues. Evaluating it can be tricky, because it can cause so many other problems in your body. Here are just a few symptoms that could be related to digestive imbalance: heartburn, gas and bloating, diarrhea or constipation, pain in your abdomen, skin problems, headaches, joint pains, fatigue, sleep issues, chronic cough, runny nose, inability to lose or gain weight, and the list goes on. This is why I often order a digestive stool test to see what is going on when someone has had chronic health problems, even if they seem unrelated to digestion.

Whether you were breastfed as an infant will affect your digestive health, too. Did you receive antibiotics? Receiving antibiotics at a very young age may affect the micro biome (the bacteria that live in your body naturally) for a long time. It can affect your current digestive health, your food reactivity, your weight, and even whether or not you have anxiety.

Digestion is complicated, and there are a ton of possibilities that could cause digestive problems including infections, parasites, bacteria, viruses, leaky gut, malabsorption, and lack of digestive enzymes, just to name a few. Once you've figured out if digestion is the root cause, you can begin to initiate healing protocols that include herbs, medication, diet, and supplements.

PRESENT TIME

The fourth factor to understand is: *where are you now?* What is happening in your life? How does your *whole body* feel? Do you feel strong? Do you feel tired, sore, weak? What have you been stressed about lately?

Think back. When did your symptoms begin? What was happening in your life at that time? Are there any circumstances that seem to help the issue, or make it worse? Who is your support system? Do you have enough support? All of these factors play a role in your health and wellness.

You may have had a health issue for only a few months, but it could have begun many years ago. For example, perhaps you had surgery on your knee when you were 25. You felt fine for years, but now, at age 60, your knee hurts all the time and is causing you back pain. Or, maybe you had Mono as a teen (commonly caused by the Epstein Barr Virus). Now, at age 50, you're having symptoms of Hashimoto's disease (fatigue, sore muscles, joint pain, depression). Hashimoto's is an autoimmune thyroid condition that is often associated with Epstein Barr Virus, in which the immune system attacks the thyroid.

Imagine that a bacteria or virus is like a little kid who wants to play hide

2nd Key: Physical Balance and Vitality

and seek. He hides under a blanket, so you don't know he's there. In this analogy, the blanket is a biofilm—a way for the bacteria or virus to hide from the immune system. By creating a biofilm, the virus uses your own body's tissue to disguise itself. The Epstein Barr virus hides in the thyroid. The immune system can't see the virus, but it sees that something is wrong with the thyroid. Since the job of the immune system is to fight foreign invaders, it begins to bang on the thyroid to try to kick it out—which causes Hashimoto's.

When you look for the root cause, you can look at your entire health history, including what you are experiencing now, and reveal a timeline of events that may show you the factors that are currently affecting your health. This can instruct your decisions about where to find answers.

Actions and Exercises for the 2nd Fundamental Finding the Root Cause

1. **Create a Health Timeline**
    a. Journal about your history. Sometimes, if you sit down and write about your earliest memories, your favorite foods, how you spent your time, and any memories of being sick as a child, you might uncover some interesting facts. Or, if you don't like to write, you can sit down with a friend and share some stories. This can become part of your health timeline.
    b. If they're available to you, you can also interview your parents or siblings about your personal health history. Everything that's ever happened to you—when you were born, vaginal delivery or Caesarean section, if you were breastfed, any adverse or traumatic childhood events, and even your vaccination history can make a huge difference in your health issues.

    c. Once you have done your research, write everything down on one document. There are even programs to create timelines (if you want to be high tech about it). You can take this to your doctor when you visit and use this for your own research.

2. **Work with an expert.** In order to locate the root source of your condition, it is helpful to seek the wisdom of an expert. A Functional Medicine doctor, a health coach or nutritionist, or a Chinese medicine practitioner would be a good place to start.

3. **Research your condition or symptoms.** Visit "Dr. Google," or buy books about your condition. But remember, though knowledge is power, you also want to leave room for miracles, and for the individuality of your own body and experience

A WORD ABOUT GENE TESTING

Understanding where you came from and your genetic history can be an important aspect of discerning your condition, but I am hesitant to universally recommend gene testing. Tests like "23 and me" can be a hindrance if you use them the wrong way. If you read the results and see that you might have an increased risk of cancer or heart disease based on your genetics, you might feel frightened that you are doomed. Many of us were raised to believe that our genetics are unchangeable. As you now know, science shows that this is not true, and we can change many elements of our genetic tendencies. *Dirty Genes*, by Dr. Lynch, gives a wonderful explanation about how we can affect our genetics.

    When I did my own genetic testing, I plugged it into a program

2nd Key: Physical Balance and Vitality

> that told me that I was at risk for heart disease, diabetes, and cancer. But when I looked more deeply at the genes, I found I had both kinds of genes: those that protect me from those diseases *and* those that make me more prone to them.
>
> Every person has redundancy of genes—there are two sides and many possibilities to every situation. The real question is whether what is imprinted in your genes will be expressed or not. Not everything in your genetics is a predetermined fate, and even if it is, you can heal it.
>
> Learning about your gene history *can* be helpful in that it can show you what you might tend toward, and you can choose to live a lifestyle that won't allow it to happen. At the same time, you want to be aware of not being too dogmatic about what you learn. People sometimes give up, or take extreme measures in reaction to the results, but as I've explained above, just because you have a certain genetic makeup does not mean that you will be condemned to a certain fate. Use the information, but keep a measure of balance in how you use or interpret it. Don't allow it to overwhelm you. Remember, information is not the same as wisdom. Working with a healer is invaluable in helping you "decode" the language of your genetic makeup.

3rd Fundamental
Cultivating Curiosity and Exploring Healing Methods

What does it mean to be curious when you're stepping into a healing process? Usually we feel awful, frightened, and angry when our bodies are in pain or feeling ill. How could curiosity play a role in getting well?

Healing When It Seems Impossible

Have you ever seen a toddler examine a new toy? He uses all of his senses to explore. He puts it in his mouth, he moves it around, he shakes it to see if it makes noise. He is full of wonder, trying to understand and make sense of this new thing in front of him. Imagine if we could approach our bodies in the same way. Imagine if we didn't always see something strange or unfamiliar as a danger, but as something to learn from?

When I encounter something new in my own body, or with a patient, I immediately see it from the perspective of a scientist—with insatiable curiosity. I want to solve the riddle. I ask questions. I research. I prescribe tests. I learn about what is happening. I find out what impacts the condition so that I can understand what might be done to change it. I approach any new issue seriously, without becoming hysterical, even when the symptoms appear frightening, because my study of the body has given me faith in its processes. (That being said, remember that you DO need to call 911 if there is an apparent emergency. **See Appendix B for a list of emergency symptoms.**)

Our bodies are always signaling where we need to pay attention. Any time you feel threatened by something happening in your body, see if you can change your approach. Become curious. Ask questions of the experts who are on your team. Explore your options for treatment. Explore your physical sensations. All treatment has its merits and can be approached from an angle of curiosity.

As much as we might like to, we usually don't go in a straight line from problem to solution in our lives. Instead, we go on a journey. Each step informs the previous and moves us forward, even if our inquiry sometimes results in a diversion. If you find yourself wanting a certain test, do it. Do everything you can. Everything that happens on your health journey has the potential to be a wondrous part of your healing. Your curiosity and interest is the gift you can give yourself, and fuels your ability to find solutions that work for you.

2nd Key: Physical Balance and Vitality

Georgia

Georgia was diagnosed with diabetes when she turned 52. When she first came to me, her intention was to heal it through natural methods. Over the course of several years, she bought books, studied online, and made many changes in her lifestyle, trying to see what would work for balancing her blood sugar naturally. She brought me the books she valued, so that I could participate in her experiments. Through her curiosity and interest, she did two things: She made me a partner in her health care, and she healed her diabetes without ever taking medication.

Healing Methods

It feels incredible when a healing modality eliminates the pain or the problem in your body. Sometimes, especially with acute injuries, that may be all that you need to do, but keep in mind with chronic or recurrent problems, there will be many other factors involved *(i.e., the six other Keys!)*. Finding balance is your ultimate goal. When you are working with the 2nd Key of physical balance, remember that you will be addressing emotional, spiritual, and lifestyle factors eventually, but you don't have to do everything at once.

Surgery and medication are often the first line of treatment for most people's issues, meaning that they are often what people first think of when they want to heal. But there are many ways you can heal. Functional medicine practices, chiropractic work, acupuncture, massage, physical therapy, hydrotherapy, biomats, supplements, and osteopathic work are just some examples of methods that can help heal your physical body.

When you choose a specific treatment modality, think of it as your friend. The treatment has your back—it is here to help you heal from something difficult and frightening. And remember, every treatment, including surgery, herbs, vitamins and massage, will have a different effect on every person.

Surgery

My first experience saving a life as a third-year medical student is precisely what made me want to go into surgery. Surgery can be absolutely miraculous. At the same time, I rarely recommend surgery for my patients unless it is necessary, because sometimes surgery will appear to fix the problem, but the energetic root of the disease may not have been addressed. If you do not deal with the root of the problem, it may arise in another way, often with more serious consequences. Creating a plan to heal from an operation, while simultaneously addressing the root issues, is the best way to fully and holistically heal.

On the positive side, surgery is an opportunity for you to make a huge shift in your body and energy. When you have surgery, you go from one physical condition to a very different physical condition *in an instant* (more or less). The key is to continue the process of healing once you have taken the initial and drastic measure.

If you must have surgery, don't put all your eggs in surgery's basket. Don't imagine that it is going to do all of the work, or that it is just something you must endure in order to be healthy. Use the surgery as springboard toward transformation, a giant step toward your health and well-being.

Don

My patient, Don, had a sudden heart attack at age 62. He was shocked, because he lived a fairly healthy lifestyle (except for his love of red wine and some stress at work) and hadn't ever considered that he might be at risk for heart disease. He had a stent placed in his coronary artery, which saved his life. After the stent was placed, he came to my office and we worked out a plan for his health, but he continued to have a lot of stress in his work and relationship. In spite of working out a plan, Don didn't want to give up his wine. He also traveled a lot for his work, so his stress really remained unchanged.

A year later, he had another episode of chest pain and his coronary artery had clogged again, which is unusual because often once you've had a stent placed and changed your lifestyle, other arteries don't get clogged within such a short time. They put another two stents in his heart.

That same year he was referred to a sleep study because we felt that his sleep might be part of the issue for his heart. We came to this conclusion because he mentioned that he was always tired in the morning, which led me to ask more questions about his sleep and discover that his wife was complaining about his snoring all the time. The studies found that he had severe sleep apnea! Once he got a CPAP machine (a specialized machine with a mask to address sleep apnea) he began sleeping much better and his heart problems improved significantly. He has been much healthier since then. In this case, the root cause of his problem was his sleep.

Of course, we can always go deeper into the root cause, depending on the patient. For Don, he felt so much better using the CPAP machine that digging deeper into the root cause of his sleep apnea did not interest him ... so we left it alone at that level. Further investigation to the root cause of his sleep apnea might have revealed that he had dietary sensitivities, or allergies, or digestive issues, or a physical obstruction in his airways.

MEDICINE

All medicine is experimental to the degree that treatments and knowledge are constantly evolving, and every person's chemistry is completely unique. For physicians, there is a certain amount of information available for almost every medicine, herb, or supplement that we can use to guide us in dispensing that item. The information includes the positive effects, some of the possible side effects, and how long it will take to be effective. What we don't know, and can never know, is how your individual body and physical chemistry will react to that medication.

Your chemistry is unique and how you respond to a prescription depends on many things, including the other medications and supplements you take, your physical sensitivity, your lifestyle, your health history, and your emotional makeup. If you've been with the same doctor for some length of time, he or she might be able to gauge how you will respond to medication based on past history and closely listening to your experiences. Yet, even this is not completely predictable.

I have found that no matter what I *think* is going on, each person responds differently to the treatment I suggest. Sometimes, in one day, I will see three or four patients with very similar physical concerns, and each is undergoing a very different treatment protocol.

I encourage my patients to listen closely to their bodies, learn how they respond to things, and to clearly report these observations to me. This enables us to work as a team for the most effective healing.

Actions and Exercises for the 3rd Fundamental
Cultivating Curiosity and Exploring Healing Methods

1. **Cultivate Curiosity by asking questions.** When you are struggling with your health, you can keep asking questions of yourself that will eventually lead you to answers:
    - What makes it better?
    - What makes it worse?
    - Is there a movement connected to the pain?
    - Is there something you can eat—or avoid eating—that makes it feel better?
    - Is it a one-time event? Does it recur?

2. **Explore alternative modalities.** If you've been trying one method of treatment and it's not working, see what else might be out there for you.

2nd Key: Physical Balance and Vitality

If you've never tried acupuncture, consider having some to see if it might help. Consider a new form of exercise to see how your body would feel with it. Or consider eating differently to see if that would make it feel better.

When you try new modalities, keep track of how they feel. Are they helpful? Does the method or treatment make sense to you? Do you feel like you are getting some relief, or a shift in symptoms?

3. **Ask yourself what emotions might be connected to your health issue.** Develop your curiosity about what the root cause might be. Could it have come from something that occurred when you were an infant? Were you abused by someone? Is your current relationship not working for you? The art of being curious is really about asking questions, and being "open" to hearing what your body has to tell you.

4th Fundamental
Build Your Relationship with Your Healthcare Provider and Healing Team

ABBY

Abby sat with her arms crossed, making it clear she was angry. It was her first visit to my office, and she spent the first part of our time together telling me that she was tired of not getting results for her various health problems when she went to see her current doctor. As I listened, I wondered, how I could help her, since she had already decided that nothing was going to work?

Abby was frustrated—and with good reason. She ate well, exercised, got enough rest, and followed her doctor's orders, but she still didn't feel well. She was doing everything right ... so why wasn't she getting better?

The healing process is often mysterious. When you see a physician, you expect results; you expect answers. The goal of the doctor is the same. We want to find out what's wrong and help you feel better—that's why we're in the business. Sometimes though, a diagnosis is not readily apparent.

In my years as a physician, there have been times that I have not found "THE ANSWER" and I am as frustrated as my patient when that happens. Fortunately, Chinese medicine gives me a different perspective and a wider range of diagnostic possibilities, and I've learned that certain conditions in the body produce health, specifically, when your hormones, immune system, and nervous system are stronger, but even with this knowledge, I cannot resolve every issue immediately.

Approaching Your Doctor or Healer

Relationship is critical to healing. We need each other, just as our bodies need each part in order to be whole. Very often, the reason that a patient isn't moving forward in their healing process is that they can't do it by themselves.

When you have a physical issue and you go see your doctor or healer, you are in a vulnerable position. You may not feel that you know enough about your body to ask the right questions and receive the information you need. Often, you feel frightened that you will have a terrible diagnosis. Even after talking to your doctor, you may still feel overwhelmed or in the dark. The important thing is to not give up—keep asking questions, keep trying to understand. Be a participant in your healing, even when you are reliant upon others.

The 2nd Key holds an interesting dichotomy. On the one hand, if you are too passive and you want someone else to just "fix" you, you will not be taking an active role in your healing, which can inhibit the process. At the same time, it is important to be able to listen, receive help, and utilize the knowledge, opinions, and expertise of others.

For a time, you may even have to "stop knowing" what you think you

2nd Key: Physical Balance and Vitality

already know about your condition in order for the healer to help.

Find a doctor or healer who will spend the time that is needed to work with you and find the appropriate treatment for your condition. Look for healers who will support your journey, rather than give you threatening messages of doom. So much of the healing journey is about the relationship between you and your healer. As the 1st Key has shown us, love is vitally important to your healing, and if you feel care from your healer, that in itself can be a powerful part of your healing process.

Just to be clear, I've met many surgeons who are caring, loving individuals and will give 100% to their patients. They may never express it, but you can tell that your health is vitally important to them. These are the doctors you want to choose; the ones you can *tell* care about you. My long-time client, Susie, recently had her uterus removed for an early intrauterine cancer. Because she'd had many abdominal surgeries over her life, she had adhesions (scar tissue) making the operation a bit more difficult. The surgeon made a video for her, showing her everything he had done, so that she could tell he had cleared the adhesions. It was obvious that her health was very important to him.

And remember, communicating effectively is a two-way street. Take the time to explore what you are feeling before you see your doctor. Write down your questions and experiences so that you are asking questions that will help you feel better. You can use the Internet, read alternative literature, or see several physicians for different opinions. For most of us, knowledge helps us to feel like we may have some control over something that often feels out of our control. When we learn more about our condition, we don't feel so helpless—in fact, we may even feel empowered. I'm aware that doctors might tell you not to use the Internet to explore your symptoms, and I do so with caution, but every single one of my patients has used the Internet to explore their condition. Denying the use of it would be unrealistic on my part.

PAM

Pam, a gentle, loving 53-year-old mother, walked into my office one day and told me she did not want to have chemotherapy and radiation for her metastatic breast cancer. She had decided to only use alternative treatments. Her plan was to use herbs, a very strict diet, and spiritual work to heal her tumors.

I became upset, because I knew her cancer was progressed and usually people need more extreme measures when they are as sick as Pam. I began to push her to use the more conventional methods. She stood her ground and firmly and gently refused to change her decision. After she left, I realized that I had tried to push her to think my way. In that moment, my fear for her had kept me from listening to her.

Pam didn't return to my office for further help, because she had chosen her path, and I hadn't supported it. Sadly, a few months later, I heard that she had died. Still, I knew that she had chosen the best treatment for her, no matter the outcome. Pam did not survive her cancer, but she approached it in the way that worked for her. She did what she felt was right, and that is the best any of us can do. Pam helped me realize that, truly, there are as many ways to approach healing as there are humans on the planet.

Actions and Exercises for the 4th Fundamental
Building Your Relationship with Your Healthcare Provider and Healing Team

1. **How to choose your doctor or healer:**
   - Choose a physician who recognizes the importance of balancing your whole body and is willing to see the significance of balancing your hormones, nervous system, and immune system (Triangle of Wellness).

- Choose a healer who practices a modality that interests you.
- Take recommendations from friends.
- Take referrals from your doctors and healers.
- Find a doctor you can trust, whom you feel listens. Then be willing to listen to them and follow their guidance.

2. **Questions for your new doctor or healer.** Depending upon your insurance, ask these questions at your initial visit. Alternatively, you can request a free or inexpensive opportunity to talk to the person who will be treating you. It is your right to see if someone works for you before you begin to invest in them.
    - Explain your health problems, and ask if they have previously handled your health problems.
    - Ask how they would approach your type of problems.
    - Be cautious when someone who says: "Yes, absolutely I will fix you," because nothing is guaranteed.
    - Ask yourself:
        - How do I feel talking to the doctor? Am I comfortable, or more agitated after seeing them?
        - Are they treating me the way I want to be treated? Do I feel better? Do I feel supported?
        - Do I feel a connection with this person?

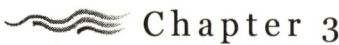 Chapter 3

3rd Key:
Choosing Your Unique Lifestyle

"The doctor of the future will give no medicines, but will interest his patients in the care of the human frame, in diet, and in the causes and prevention of disease."
—THOMAS EDISON

"The secret of change is to focus all of your energy, not on fighting the old, but on building the new."
—SOCRATES

DISCOVERING WHO YOU ARE

We want a cure that's sexy. We want something quick that takes care of everything. We want "How-To" guides—to know that by doing *this*, we will accomplish *that* … But "how-to" doesn't work the same way for every person, and instructions don't account for the uniqueness of your individual body.

Lifestyle is all about discovery. Yes, there are some guidelines we all can follow, but discovering your unique lifestyle means learning about yourself. How do you enjoy life? How do you give to yourself? What is unique about your needs, and what works for *you*?

3rd Key: Choosing Your Unique Lifestyle

We tend to devote most of our time and energy to Lifestyle—the 3rd Key. It's how we care for ourselves every day, and it's where we have the most actionable control. Whether it's eating ice cream when we are sad, or having an intense workout after we've had an argument, we turn to Lifestyle when we seek emotional, mental, and physical support, and it often quickly helps us feel better.

Lifestyle is the most physically active of the 7 Keys. It includes your sleep, how you exercise, how and what you eat, the supplements you take, and other self-care habits and choices. Lifestyle also includes your attitude. It is deeply influenced by weather, the environment, and the seasons.

You can find a tremendous amount of information and how-to guides about improving your lifestyle in the world and online, and the choices can feel overwhelming. What we are going to address in this chapter is the greatest challenge: How do you discern which actions *you can take* and what changes *you can make* to improve your own life and health. What are the right choices *for you*?

PHYSICAL STRENGTH = EMOTIONAL STRENGTH

One of the premises of this book is that everything is connected. By doing one thing, you can impact your whole system. Therefore, by working on your lifestyle you can indeed change other areas of imbalance, which is why it's so powerful. This means that what you eat, how you exercise, and how much sleep you get will also affect your emotional well-being. Sometimes, it's easier to deal with the lifestyle aspects of our lives than process emotional elements. Since your physical body is home to your emotions and spirit, when you take care of your body, you are naturally also attending to every part of you. It's like healing yourself *from the outside in*.

On the other hand, if your lifestyle is poor, and you eat foods that don't agree with your body, or you don't get enough sleep or exercise, it will be stressful to your body. Stress affects your mind, your hormones, and your energy levels. Poor lifestyle choices can cause a decreased ability to cope with painful emotions, make decisions, and find those feel-good moments. Taking care of the physical elements of your health creates greater emotional stability, which also makes changing your lifestyle easier. Everything is connected.

Fundamentals of the 3rd Key
Choosing Your Unique Lifestyle

The 3rd Key is about embarking on a journey to discover who you are, what you need, and how to be in the world physically on a daily basis. Your foundation is already strong through the work that you've done with the 1st and the 2nd Keys. You've strengthened your relationship with your body and the healing process (1st Key), and have gained tools to support and balance your body on the most fundamental levels (2nd Key). With those skills in hand, you are now ready to look more deeply at your habits, what triggers you, and what makes you feel good so you can make the necessary adjustments to your daily life.

The 3rd Key grounds and activates your healing process, and allows you to approach the less-tangible elements of the final Keys with more clarity and stability.

Below are essential concepts to help you navigate your lifestyle choices. The focus of Lifestyle in this book is to take you through steps that will reveal your own specific lifestyle needs so you can respond, now and in the future, in the best possible way for your body and health. The how-to in this chapter discusses how you can learn to access your own truth when it comes to living your exceptionally individual and dynamic life.

3rd Key: Choosing Your Unique Lifestyle

1st Fundamental: Preventive Health Care
Most people don't pay attention to their well-being until they are in a health crisis. How can you make your own well-being as important as the health of your loved ones? What might motivate you, and create an impetus for staying healthy and avoiding or minimizing sickness? Choosing to value your good health ideal is so much better than waiting for an illness or trauma to motivate healthy actions and attitudes.

2nd Fundamental: Discovering Your Unique Path
Balance is unique to each individual. What is healthy for one person may not work for another. The process of living a healthy lifestyle requires recognizing what your body needs and acting upon that understanding.

3rd Fundamental: Reduce the Noise
"Noise" impacts the quiet, easy flow of energy in our bodies, and is extremely pervasive. Stemming from the foods we eat, the toxins in our environment, and our daily stressors, they create a loud racket and translate into inflammation in the body. This noise is the cause of many chronic physical issues, and it can also affect our ability to hear the quieter signals our body is sending us. The best (and only) way to clear the noise is to work to remove the triggers. You can't truly know how something is impacting your life unless you remove it; it's only in the contrast that you can know how something is affecting you.

4th Fundamental: Moderation
Moderation is the central theme to a healthy life in both Chinese and Western medicine. Practicing moderation in all elements of your life, including work, food, drink, sex, exercise, and sleep, establishes a stable foundation that affects not only your body, but also your mind, spirit, and emotions. Too much or too little of *anything* can cause an imbalance

in your energy and affect your mental and physical health.

5th Fundamental: Stagnation and Flexibility
Life requires flexibility—an ability to move and change with ever-evolving circumstances. And, a big part of good health means actively mixing things up. Being stuck in a rut, even if the choice was originally a healthy one, can lead to stagnation and ultimately poor health.

6th Fundamental: Attitude
Attitude may seem to relate more to your emotional well-being, but in the 7 Keys, attitude is directly related to your lifestyle because there is such a decisive and active quality about it. At the same time, eating well, exercise, and supplements—the cornerstones of the 3rd Key—naturally improve your attitude. So your lifestyle supports and complements your attitude, and your attitude boosts and motivates your lifestyle, essentially creating a circuit of healthy energy.

1st Fundamental
Preventive Health Care

CHARLOTTE
Charlotte is extremely healthy, active, and health conscious. A few years ago, her husband had severe lymphoma. He underwent chemotherapy, a bone marrow transplant, and had to spend months in the hospital. While he was in the hospital, Charlotte woke up every morning at 5 a.m. to be at his bedside and to make sure that everything was going as well as possible. For months she was under unremitting, severe stress as her husband lingered on life support. Her ability to remain healthy and strong while she was caring for her husband was

due to the fact that she had previously been taking such excellent care of her body.

What Is Preventive Medicine?

For countless reasons, we tend to suppress, ignore, or deny symptoms until a problem has progressed and forces us to seek medical attention. Receiving physical support is often necessary when symptoms are more advanced, but *the imperative of healing and being healthy* is to find out what you can do to create more balance in your body *before you get sick.*

The use of conventional Western medical tests to determine your risk for various conditions is generally covered by health insurance as "preventive medicine." These include standard blood tests, colonoscopy, mammograms, testing cholesterol levels, and pap smears, to name a few. In truth, these tests are more "early detection" than preventive because they only show when there is already a problem. Having said that, they are useful, and can hopefully detect a problem early enough, before the disease has progressed too far.

If you have a family history of a particular disease, or you've been told that you are at risk for something, talk to your doctor and set up a plan of what you can do to stay healthy. At some point in each person's life, imbalances in the body begin to become apparent. It's our job to pay attention to those signals. Be as determined to stay healthy as you are to heal from an illness. That is preventive medicine!

Making the Leap: Olympians of Health

Most health issues have deep roots. Something was off balance for a long time and we weren't paying attention, or we didn't recognize the signs, or it may even have begun in childhood without our knowledge. Suddenly, we are dealing with a crisis. Every one of my patients who has a serious illness can tell me the moment in their lives when they began to feel that they needed to do something different. The problem was, they either didn't know what they needed to do, or they didn't really recognize the importance of making a change.

Change can be scary, because it usually means leaping into the unknown. We wonder what's going to happen. What does the future hold? How can I embrace change?

What if change occurred at a different pace? What if you could create an impetus for change when nothing is obviously wrong? We all struggle with paying attention to our own needs, since there are so many other people and details to take care of in our lives. What if we could make our health a number one priority—no matter what was going on and no matter how we felt—even when we are *not* sick?

The trick is to remember that change by choice is always faster and more effective than change by necessity or trauma—especially when it comes to healing. And when you help yourself, you are also helping your loved ones—financially, emotionally, physically, mentally ... in every way!

Each of us has a font of energy inside that we can tap into. The best way to find this energy is to allow yourself to feel cared for. This doesn't mean hoarding time or resources; it's about actively participating in your health and seeing the benefit of that. Find what makes you feel nurtured and supported. Find what you can do to feel better. When you take charge, you'll feel more in control, confident, less stressed, and happier.

Olympic athletes don't just train right before a competition; their training influences every part of their lives. They are constantly thinking about and moving toward their goal. Their diligence, discipline, and totality of focus is what creates their expertise. They work to develop muscle memory that allows them to achieve mastery, so something that was once difficult becomes second nature through practice. Their totality gives them grace and allows them to triumph.

We all can be Olympians of our own health. It requires focus, discipline, and diligence—qualities that we can work on. Changing your lifestyle and

3rd Key: Choosing Your Unique Lifestyle

habits without the push of illness means working to create a strong awareness and connection to your body. If you feel something happening in your body, check it out early, before the symptoms become extreme. If something already feels bad, get it checked out, ask questions, do your research. Take control of your health.

Life is unpredictable. We never know when something will happen that will challenge us to our limits. By taking care of your body when you feel healthy, you will be better able to stay healthy in times of stress and recover more quickly when you do become unwell. It's like having savings in your physical bank account.

Actions for the 1st Fundamental Preventive Health Care

1. **Prevention—Do It Before You Get Sick!**
   - Take the time to put together your healing team, including acupuncturists, nutritionists, chiropractors, trainers, etc. *before* you get sick. This will give you more body awareness, and allow experts to be acquainted with your body. In that way, you are more likely to discover a serious illness before it becomes serious, or avoid it altogether.
   - Find practitioners who will support your life and lifestyle, who listen to you, and with whom you can communicate.
   - See an integrative medical doctor or functional medicine doctor.
   - Prioritize your lifestyle health: diet, exercise, sleep, and stress level.
   - Keep up with early detection testing (as indicated).

2. **Review Your Genetics**

   If you have a family history of a particular health issue, find ways to live preventively. You can usually find lifestyle options that will help prevent most genetic imbalances from occurring. For example, if you have a family history of heart disease, you can do things that will make you less prone to the problem: begin a program of eating a Mediterranean diet, exercise regularly, and engage in active stress management to ensure that you can keep yourself healthy.

   It's never too late to start a lifestyle overhaul. Do research on your genetics and then create a plan to prevent the problems. It should be noted: this is something that can be helpful to do with a practitioner who understands this process, such as a nutritionist, or doctor who understands genetics.

3. **Make Sure That You Feel Financially Secure to Take Care of Your Health**
   - Plan for it financially.
   - Make sure that you have coverage for serious health issues (health insurance).
   - Prioritize supplements, medication, and other modalities in your budget (understanding that it will save you money, expenses, and loss of work in the long run!).

4. **Create a Schedule to "Pay Yourself First"**

   People often tell me they don't have time to be more committed to exercising or eating a certain way. If you don't "make" time, you certainly will never have it. In the financial world, we are famously told to "pay ourselves first," in other words, to put aside a reserve of money for emergencies and savings before paying all the bills.

   Usually, about 10 percent of our gross income is recommended to set

3rd Key: Choosing Your Unique Lifestyle

aside. You can do the same thing with your lifestyle.

Create a schedule with time dedicated to take care of yourself. No matter how busy your life is, give yourself a little time. Even if it's only ten minutes during the day to do a yoga pose or jumping jacks, or five minutes to meditate, make a start, and it will begin to make a difference.

2nd Fundamental
Discovering Your Unique Path

Why do we each have a different response to the same illness? Why will one person live five years with the same disease that kills another in six months?

Recently, I had several patients with similar symptoms. All three women experienced severe anxiety, nausea, upset stomach, stomachaches, and heartburn, but the cause and the resolution of their symptoms was different for each one. All three women benefited from receiving acupuncture, yet each woman required a different approach to healing.

THE ISSUES AND THEIR BACKSTORIES

JANIE

When Janie turned 59, she began worrying that she would die soon, because her mother had died when she was 60. That same year, Janie's husband had a heart attack. Janie began to develop stomach problems and felt like she was no longer in control of her life. According to Chinese medicine, the stomach is connected to the emotion of worry. Janie had always been a spiritual person. She had used spiritual methods to heal from illnesses in the past, but those tools didn't work with her current problems. Over the years, her hormones had shifted and her eating habits were making her hormones worse.

Janie normally did not eat for two hours after she woke up in the morning. Her anxiety caused her cortisol levels to be high, and when she missed breakfast, her cortisol went even higher. She compounded this issue by drinking coffee on an empty stomach. Coffee drives the blood sugar lower, which in her case caused nausea. Finally, drinking coffee on an empty stomach gave her heartburn.

The Solution
Caffeine and Breakfast

Janie quit drinking coffee and started having breakfast with protein to raise her blood sugar and help stabilize her hormones in the mornings. This simple change reduced her anxiety throughout the day, which began to alleviate her stomachaches. She then realized that her stomachaches had been contributing to her anxiety, so as body began to relax, her mind did as well.

Marie

Marie was 35 years old and had uncontrollable anxiety. She was recently married and wanted to have a baby. She was the oldest child, and her family was quite traditional, so there was a lot of pressure to do everything right, in the proper order, at the proper time. Before she came to see me she had not made the connection between how her emotions were affecting her body. She was so anxious that she could not eat, and felt nauseated, which made her feel more anxious. It was a vicious cycle that kept getting worse.

The Solution
Supplements and Relaxation

In addition to acupuncture, Marie began to take supplements to raise her serotonin levels. As she recognized the connection between her body, mind, and emotions, she learned some exercises to relax her mind in order to lessen her anxiety.

3rd Key: Choosing Your Unique Lifestyle

SUSAN

Susan was 63 when she started to have severe stomachaches. She had been borderline anxious for years, but had learned to cope with her anxiety, so it took her by surprise when her stomach got so bad that she couldn't eat anything. She felt more and more sick. Her doctors gave her every kind of test, but they could not find any answers for her problems. Susan had always been a thin woman, but was becoming even thinner. Within the three weeks before she came to see me, she had lost 15 pounds.

From the angle of Chinese medicine, Susan's stomach was rebelling against her. She couldn't keep any food down. The nausea was making her anxious because she knew she couldn't get better if she didn't eat. Each time she ate, the cycle of anxiety, stomachaches, and being unable to keep food down became more vicious.

The Solution

Diet

Healing for Susan involved healing her stomach so she could begin to tolerate food again, and then balancing her hormones. She needed acupuncture before she could even tolerate food. Then she began a very special diet to slowly increase her tolerance of food. Within three weeks she was able to eat almost normally again.

HONOR YOUR INDIVIDUALITY

You are completely unique—your biology and history guarantee it. Your skin, your eyes, your fingerprints, the way you react, how you think, how you were raised, your emotional makeup—all are completely unique to you. In the same way, your responses to foods, exercise, supplements, and healing modalities have a particular connection to you.

Pay attention to your responses. How do you feel, emotionally, physically, and mentally when you eat a particular food, or exercise in a certain way? Are there any patterns you can detect? Are there certain times of the day, or certain experiences that cause you to feel more irritable, more tired, more angry, or more mentally awake? All of these factors are clues into how you might address changes to your lifestyle in the most beneficial manner.

Just because an exercise regime or a diet has miraculous effect for a friend does not mean that it will work for you. Some people thrive on a raw vegan diet, while others feel completely malnourished and fatigued. Some digestive systems cannot tolerate uncooked vegetables, while other bodies have a harder time breaking down meats and fats.

As you are exploring different lifestyle elements, treat the exploration like an adventure. You are discovering—or re-discovering—your responses and your likes and dislikes. You are on a journey of getting to know yourself anew, and all great discoveries require devotion to exploration. Listen to your body and honor your individuality.

Become a Scientist (like Einstein!)

People often approach their lifestyle mathematically: If I do *this*, I will achieve *this*. Yet the equations for each person are different, and so the best way to achieve the desired outcome is to approach your health scientifically, like a scientist—a wonderfully mad scientist! What is going to happen to your emotions, your body, and your energy if you stop eating sugar? How does your energy change throughout the day ... throughout the year ... or with the change of seasons? When a challenge becomes an interesting puzzle to solve rather than an aggravation, your whole perspective and experience can shift.

Progress happens when we push the limits of what we already know. By activating our inner explorer or inner scientist, we begin to open doors that could not otherwise be found. You might begin to notice that certain foods make your body feel especially good. You might notice that after eating lunch you get really sleepy. As you notice these things, just play with changing one or two habits a month to see how you feel. You can keep a little notebook of

3rd Key: Choosing Your Unique Lifestyle

your experiments so that you can keep track of what has changed.

Follow your intuition and the clues that life gives you. If you find a supplement, or read about something that seems like it would work, try it. Maybe you consistently forget to take certain supplements—perhaps this is not the right thing for you to take. Maybe you stop eating dairy, and discover that your nose clears up for the first time in forever. Give yourself permission to try things that may seem completely outside your comfort zone.

Remember to have patience with the process when you are experimenting. It can take 2-4 weeks to really feel the results of a change that you've made. Stick with it! If you're not seeing immediate results, give yourself other rewards for your hard work and dedication. At the same time, don't continue to do something if it's not making a difference. After 2-4 weeks, if you don't feel a change, ask yourself, "Does my body want this?"

You can't do everything all at once. Start with something simple. My unique lifestyle has evolved over years. I've changed how I eat, how I sleep, and how I exercise many times. It's evolving all the time. Each time I make a change, I can see what works and what doesn't work for me.

Actions and Exercises for the 2nd Fundamental Discovering Your Unique Path

1. **Eat Protein for Breakfast**
   One thing that *most* people can benefit from is eating a high protein breakfast within one hour of waking up. Your hormones will be more balanced from eating breakfast, and you'll feel better right away.

2. **Experiment**
   - **Add one healthy item to your diet.** Adding something new, rather than removing something, is preferable for most people. For example, you can add one large portion of green vegetables to your diet every day.
   - **Change one food that you eat a lot.** If you eat bread often, simply removing that from your diet will require creativity and exploration into new and different food options.
   - **Change up your exercise habits.** Start with something that you like to do. Find an activity that you've always wanted to try and go do it. Dance. Try Tai Chi. Take an urban hike. Join a meet-up group. The benefits will probably go way beyond your physical health.
   - **Go to bed by 10 pm.** According to Chinese medicine it is best to go to sleep by 10 or 10:30 pm and to sleep until around 7 am. In that time, the organs repair, process, and replenish your energy, so you can awake ready for the day!

3rd Key: Choosing Your Unique Lifestyle

3. **Keep a Journal**
   - Keep a journal of your experiences as you explore your lifestyle.
   - Have a section for each area of experimentation: diet, exercise, supplements, sleep, etc.
   - Write down all the changes you are making, and include any noticeable differences in:
     - your physical appearance
     - your energy
     - your emotions
     - your mental clarity/concentration
     - your digestive function—such as changes in bowel movements, appetite, gas/bloating, or abdominal pain
   - When you find what makes you feel better, stick with it!

4. **Building New Habits**

   The challenge to creating a new lifestyle habit is that it takes 90 days to really establish. If you don't do something new for at least 90 days, it might not become embedded. For most people, 90 days can feel like a lifetime when you're trying to change something!

   In order to overcome this initial obstacle, I usually commit to trying something new for a couple of weeks in order to decide if it's good for me. Once I know that I like it, or see that it's working, I step into committing to it as a lifestyle change. For example, when I first started Barre class a couple of years ago, I went a few times in the course of two weeks. I realized that I liked it, so I began to work it into my schedule regularly.

   Don't just do something one time and decide it's not for you. Below are some possible ways to begin a new habit.

Diet
- If you are a person who skips breakfast, try eating breakfast every morning for a week and notice how you feel.
- Without changing anything else in your diet, try adding lots more vegetables. Make half your plate low-carb vegetables (green vegetables are mostly low-carb) every day for two weeks and see how you feel.
- Basic good diet habits include not eating any processed foods. Can you eliminate one processed food that you like a lot (like white sugar) for a month and see how you feel?

Exercise
- Start with one new exercise that you haven't tried before, even if you usually exercise a lot. Try something new, like a yoga class, or Pilates.
- Do something you love.
- Have fun when you exercise. Join a team or a dance class.
- According to Chinese medicine principles, certain exercises are most beneficial at certain times of the year:
    - In winter you want to do more gentle building exercises like yoga.
    - In spring, try running and doing more cardio—push your breathing.
    - In summer, exercise should be outdoors during the cooler times of day.
    - Late summer you want to incorporate more weights and strengthening exercises into your routine.
    - Fall: include more breath work with your regular exercise.
- Break it up into doable projects (20 minutes, 30 minutes, at home, etc.).

- Remember that you are giving to yourself and you are helping your whole body and your whole health.
- Find a partner

Find at Least One Support Person

Finding someone who encourages you, and who you feel accountable to, can really help as you are trying to change your lifestyle habits.
- Find a partner or buddy who will do this with you, or find someone who is willing to support you as you make changes in your life.
- If you cannot think of anyone to support you, check my private Facebook support group, "Healing When It Seems Impossible."

3rd Fundamental
Reduce the Noise

"Let thy food be thy medicine and thy medicine be thy food."
—Hippocrates (460-377 B.C.)

Thomas

Thomas quit eating gluten when his wife was diagnosed with celiac disease—a severe allergic reaction to gluten—and she had to give it up. Thomas himself was not experiencing problems with gluten as far as he knew, but he promised his wife he would quit so that it would be easier for her.

Two weeks later, his wife asked Thomas if he noticed that he was no longer depressed. She thought that it was maybe because he had stopped eating gluten. He hadn't noticed, but immediately he decided to test her theory by eating a pizza. The next day he was so depressed he could hardly function. Since then,

Thomas maintains a gluten-free diet. Even though his digestion does not seem to be affected by gluten, he realized just how much his emotions are affected by it.

Many of us live with symptoms and don't really question them; they become a part of our everyday experience. We go about our lives and do all kinds of things in certain patterns. Often these patterns reinforce the symptoms that we're experiencing. Simply by changing the patterns of what we're doing (how we eat, what we think, etc.) we can begin to reduce the "noise" and hear better what our body is saying.

Most of us are not completely aware of all the noise in our everyday lives. It's not just the actual noise all around us—from cars to machinery, to TV, to other people—*our lives and bodies are also filled with "noise."* Our minds are constantly active, thinking and worrying. Our emotions can seize us and make it hard to "hear" anything else. And our physical bodies are constantly working to process everything we go through, including the food we eat, the emotions we experience, the physical activity that we are doing (or are not doing), as well as the vital acts of beating our hearts, breathing our breath, and regulating our temperature. You can imagine then, that when we clutter our bodies with food that is difficult to process, the noise becomes louder.

Meditation was created to help clear the mind and emotions. The premise is that by focusing on something simple, like your breath or a mantra, you can slow down and clear your mind, which heightens your ability to think and act. In a similar way, when you cleanse you body of toxins and allergens you help clear the noise so that you can actually hear what your body is trying to say.

Below, I have recommended an intensive elimination diet, because it's the best way to truly see how food is affecting your health. In the healing process, there's a time where you have to be really strict. This step can be difficult for some people—but it's so important. You've already made a big commitment by reading this book; why not go all in?

3rd Key: Choosing Your Unique Lifestyle

Eventually, I advise that everyone do this diet in order to reduce the noise in their bodies, but if it feels like too much to take on at first, just change one thing. Start with something simple. Do it consistently for two weeks, and see how you feel. The simplest thing to change is an eating habit, but you can also try going to bed at the same time every night, or eat a light breakfast if you normally don't. You could even try meditating if you don't usually meditate. Pay attention to your energy level, your sleep patterns, your skin, your digestion, your mood, any joint pain, headaches, or any physical changes that you experience. Keep a log of these observations.

Actions and Exercises for the 3rd Fundamental
Reduce the Noise

1. **Elimination Diet**

   There are several ways to do an elimination diet. The idea is to eliminate all possible triggers for three weeks and then slowly add one item at a time back into your diet and see how you feel.

   I'm going to describe the most simple and strict way to do an elimination diet. This allows the greatest potential to see what is working for your body or not.

   Being on the elimination diet for a few weeks can lead to changes in your taste buds and a greater level of sensitivity about which foods cause changes or symptoms in your body. Symptoms that are currently a problem are likely to improve during the elimination diet, although there can be an initial period of worsening symptoms because of detoxification.

   After the initial phase of the elimination diet, where you remove all of the trigger foods, there is a reintroduction phase. As the avoided foods are carefully brought back into an eating plan, patients can see which foods trigger the symptoms they experienced prior to the elimination diet. Overall, after the elimination diet, patients will notice they are much more in touch with their body's response to food.

Here is a list of all the foods to eliminate for three weeks and foods to eat

Foods to stay away	Foods to eat
(If you feel like this is too much, then just stay away from gluten and dairy for three weeks and see how that feels.)	Game meats (lamb, rabbit, bison)
	Poultry
	Fish
	Dairy alternatives
	Gluten free whole grains (quinoa, amaranth, millet, teff, wild rice, brown rice)
Dairy	
Gluten	
Sugar, including alcohol	Legumes (except peanuts)
Chocolate	Healthy oils
Eggs	Seeds
Peanuts	Nuts (except peanuts)
Corn	Vegetables
Soy	Fruits

After three weeks of eating the elimination diet you will be ready to introduce foods back into your diet.

3rd Key: Choosing Your Unique Lifestyle

2. **Here Is How You Reintroduce Foods to Your Diet**

   To help identify potential problem foods once the Elimination Diet has been completed, foods that seemed associated with symptoms ("challenge foods") should be reintroduced into the diet, one at a time in two-day intervals. See above foods to avoid. Start with the food that you missed the most during the elimination diet. Many people start testing with dairy, or gluten …

   a. On the first day of the reintroduction phase, choose whatever food you missed or craved the most, or choose the food you had previously eaten most often. The order of which foods you reintroduce first is not critical.

   b. Eat a generous amount of that food throughout for two days (two or three average-size portions), while continuing to eat the other foods on the Elimination Diet. During that day and the next, observe your body to see if you feel any return of old symptoms, or if you develop new ones.

   c. If there is no reaction to the food during this two-day period, keep that food in the food plan. Stay on the elimination diet otherwise for two days, so now you're on day four of observing. On day four, reintroduce a second food. Watch for any new symptoms on Day Four and Five. If there is no reaction, keep that food in the diet and add the third challenge food, and so on.

   If any food provokes symptoms, stop eating that food immediately, go back to the baseline elimination diet until the symptoms clear, then reintroduce the next food.

   d. After testing all of the challenge foods, try the problem foods again (the ones that made your symptoms return) using the same procedure (one day of eating the food and noting symptoms during the following two-day period).

   After you've done the elimination diet, you will know more about how your body feels with various foods. Then you can decide how you want to live. Knowledge is power, and when you know what your body reacts to, you have the power to choose how to live.

The whole point of this intensive exercise is to learn about your body and to feel as good as possible.

4th Fundamental
Moderation

Now that you have worked to reduce the noise in your body, the next step is to find how you can maintain that balance. When it comes to your lifestyle, the key to balance is *moderation*.

In Chapter 5 we learned about *jing*—your life force energy. You receive jing when you are born, from your parents, but the other part of *jing* is connected to your lifestyle. It is how you spend your life energy. The idea is that you are born with a certain amount of energy, and over the course of your life—depending upon how you live—you restore or deplete your energy, like a bank account. If you overdo food, exercise, sex, alcohol, or work, you will deplete your essence. In the same way, if you live your life focused upon restoring your energy, your energy will be stronger.

The central theme of Chinese medicine is to find a way to live in the center, which means exercising moderation in all aspects of living. Moderation in lifestyle choices does not guarantee health, but it can safeguard against imbalances from other areas of your life where we have less immediate and direct control.

Imagine a pendulum, which swings from one side to the other. At one side of the pendulum is being hyper-strict about your diet and lifestyle with no tolerance for little indulgences, the upturns of life, or simple play. At the

3rd Key: Choosing Your Unique Lifestyle

other side of the pendulum is overindulging in sweets, alcohol and carbs, working too many hours, avoiding exercise, not getting enough sleep. Your eventual goal is to find your own center between the two, where you don't feel fanatic about your lifestyle but you are confidently and consistently practicing healthy lifestyle choices and awareness of what is good for you.

NOTE ABOUT ALLERGIES

The only time that the practice of moderation cannot apply is in regard to allergies or addictions. In Chinese medicine, an allergy occurs because the body's ability to protect itself has become distorted, which causes the immune system to overreact to something. Sometimes we are born with allergies, and sometimes we acquire an allergy, but the only way to deal with a true food allergy is through staying away from that food completely.

PLAY WITH YOUR EDGES

Moderation is a process of becoming aware. Once your body is in balance and you are feeling healthy, you can do an 80/20 or 85/15 plan of following your diet and exercise path. 80–85% of the time you maintain discipline with your diet and exercise—eating the right foods for your body and exercising regularly. 15-20% of the time you can indulge a little, and eat those treats you find that you have to avoid.

I used to eat perfectly five days a week, and on the weekends not so much. At this point in my life, because of my food sensitivities, I have to be more disciplined throughout the week. Once or twice a week I will do one thing that is not so healthy for me, like have a sugary snack or a margarita.

If you are sick or feeling bad, you have to be 100% disciplined on your healing path. See it as a gift you are giving yourself. Until your body is more balanced, it is not the time to practice moderation. Instead, it is time to practice totality. Every time you use restraint and choose healthy foods, every time you exercise, you are choosing a better life and future for yourself.

And when your body is healthy, you have room to play with your edges. It's OK to push the envelope a little and see how much can you do. As you have journeyed on this path thus far, you're going to realize where you can't overindulge as much as you once did. It's your body's way of helping you to be more balanced and healthy. The more you look at what you're reacting to, the more you want to give your body what makes it feel the best.

Actions and Exercises for the 4th Fundamental Moderation

1. **Review Your Lifestyle**

    On a scale of 1-10, where do you feel you are doing things either excessively or not at all? One (1) being not at all, and ten (10) is thinking about or doing something all the time.

    - How much do you exercise?
    - How much time you spend sitting each day?
    - How much sugar do you eat?
    - How much caffeine do you drink?
    - How much alcohol do you drink?
    - How many hours of sleep do you get each night?
    - What time do you get up in the night?
    - How many portions of vegetables do you eat each day?
    - How much water do you drink?

3rd Key: Choosing Your Unique Lifestyle

- How stressful is your job (1 being not stressful, 10 being extremely stressful)

Next, think about how you might change one thing—perhaps add five minutes to your exercise routine today. Or, go to bed ten minutes earlier. Or, set your alarm to get up a few minutes earlier.

2. **Mindfulness**

   Take one thing that you do every day, and slow it waaaaaay down. Let's say you make a cup of tea every morning: slow down your movements so that it takes up to 30 seconds for your arm to move one foot. Do the slow motion exercise for two minutes a day. When you slow down your movements, you become aware of the elements involved in your behavior. It allows you to be aware of when you are hungry, when you are taking something just for the heck of it, and when you really want it. If you do this while eating, chewing a bite, and putting your fork down before the next bite, you will notice when you are full, and won't eat as much.

5th Fundamental
Stagnation and Flexibility

Life is uncertain, so our routines give us comfort, predictability, and a sense of safety. For many of us, those daily actions keep our lives on track, but when routines become inflexible, or when they cause us to stop paying attention and we go on "autopilot," they can cause stagnation in our energy. Routines are not unhealthy, but sometimes we become so accustomed to a certain routine that we may not even be aware of its effects.

Pain is energy that is not moving. Therefore, stagnation is the root of many health concerns in Chinese medicine. When energy does not circulate freely through the body, you can develop pain, fatigue, digestive problems, tumors, and other symptoms.

According to Chinese medicine, the liver regulates the smooth movement of energy through your body, so stagnation often originates there. The liver also stores the blood *(the spleen makes the blood, and the liver stores it)*, regulates the eyes and menstrual cycles, and helps you accomplish things. It rules the emotions of anger and frustration.

One way our energy can become stuck or stagnant is when we hold onto our anger. Holding onto a negative emotion may cause tension in our neck and shoulders, or menstrual problems such as PMS, or severe cramps. Many health problems can develop from stuck anger in our bodies, so it is vitally important to find ways to release our anger (this will be discussed more in Chapter 5). Aerobic exercise is probably the best way to move out stuck anger in the body.

Maintaining flexibility can ultimately help you stay young, vibrant, and less stuck physically and mentally. Like moving water that is trapped or constricted, when your energy does not move smoothly, it can stagnate and become unhealthy. Just one small lifestyle change, like laughing more often, can help you see everything differently. Something as small as changing the route you drive to work one morning can release a stagnant flow. Go to a different restaurant for lunch, or start a new healthful habit, like eating more vegetables or walking an extra ten minutes a day.

The willingness to experiment and try something new or different in response to the ways our body is changing, will loosen trappings or constrictions. The willingness to "think outside the box," to be curious and enthusiastic about discovery is so necessary to moving and bending with the ebb and flow of life.

Your Body Is Your Own School

In my experience, the ability to adapt quickly under stressful circumstances

3rd Key: Choosing Your Unique Lifestyle

is a reasonably accurate definition of good health. In my years practicing medicine, I have met countless amazing people, and the people who inspire me the most are those who see life and death as an opportunity to grow and learn. This is something we understandably forget when we become sick: we tend to focus on what we *don't* want. As the poet, philosopher, and cancer survivor Mark Nepo stated, "We tend to make what's in the way, *the way.*"

So how do we, as adults, reach a place of flexibility and adaptability, especially in terms of our health? We can understand that our body is one of the best teachers in life. All of our experiences—good, bad, and indifferent—are important, and are an opportunity to learn something new. Every step of the healing process is a part of your journey. Every step can be an adventure. By trusting your experiences, and feeling that they are helping you *learn*, by not judging them, as children don't judge, you can learn to feel more flexible, positive, and adaptable in your life.

Actions and Exercises for the 5th Fundamental Stagnation and Flexibility

1. **Practice Flexibility**

    Do a few stretches every morning: gentle stretches that improve your physical flexibility will also improve your emotional flexibility. If you feel like you're too stiff to stretch, try just very gentle stretches every day for five minutes (that don't induce pain) and within one week you will notice that you're more flexible.

    First thing in the morning, do gentle stretching—not pushing beyond your limits, but pushing to the edge. Lift arms above your head, stretch your legs out long, and roll from side to side.

2. **Get Unstuck**

   Think about one area of your life where you feel stuck. Perhaps you feel like you can't move forward on a project, or you're having trouble losing weight. What action can you take to change your experience of feeling stuck? Remember that small, seemingly unrelated actions can help you with changing. Here is a short list of ideas:
   - If you feel stuck with your diet, change one thing that you eat.
   - Visit a new neighborhood.
   - Call a friend you haven't talked to in a long time.
   - Clean a closet or file drawer you haven't even looked at in ages.
   - Drive a new way to work.
   - Go out to dinner in a nice restaurant alone.
   - Try a new exercise class.
   - Eat something you've never eaten before.
   - Plan a trip to a foreign country.

3. **Spring "Cleaning"**

   While you don't have to wait for springtime to change a habit, it is the best time of year to initiate a big change. It is the time of year of the liver, which is the organ responsible for getting things done, and it's when sap starts flowing, winter thaws out, and flowers are blooming. I always host a cleanse during this time of year because it's such a great time to make changes. One reason I believe that many New Year's resolutions don't succeed is because January is the middle of winter, when the body's energy systems are in hibernation mode. Energy is lower at that time of year, and we aren't cut out to cleanse or make big changes then. This is part of my seasonal approach to healing, to use the time of year in an optimal way to support it.

   Twice a year, in the spring and in the fall, I host a cleanse. This is a time when you can reboot your body's system so that you can start the season out fresh. It can be used in any way you like; you can just follow a cleansing diet and take the supplements that support liver detox, digestion and kidneys. Or you can use it to review your entire life.

Being willing to change a habit at least once a year, even if it's just a temporary change, gives us more resilience and flexibility, which is an essential part of maintaining health and illness prevention.

6th Fundamental
Attitude

"There are only two ways to live your life. One is as though nothing is a miracle. The other is as though everything is a miracle."
—ALBERT EINSTEIN

AIKIDO

When I was an ER doctor in Seattle, I worked the night shift because I was attending acupuncture school during the day. One night, an extremely intoxicated patient came into the ER with a broken front tooth. He was a small man, only about 5 feet tall, and weighed about 100 pounds. I had the job of getting his tooth back into his mouth. Often, when a tooth is fractured, it can be reattached, so I was trying to help him, but he attacked me with all of his might. His attack frightened me so much that I wanted to hit him back! Instead, the guards were nearby and they rushed to protect me.

After that night, I decided to start taking Aikido classes. Aikido is a Japanese martial art, a non-violent technique where you use the energy of an attacker to defend yourself in a non-violent way *and* protect the attacker from injury. I had many intoxicated, belligerent, and potentially dangerous patients throughout my experience in the ER, and I hoped that by learning some basic moves in Aikido I would learn to defend myself without hurting my attacker.

Within one month, I stopped having violent patients! I never again had a patient attack me. At that point in my Aikido lessons, I hadn't even learned how to defend myself, I had only learned to bow and roll over. It seemed that Aikido had empowered me to feel stronger and more centered so that those potentially dangerous patients no longer saw me as a target. I still had patients who were drunk or high on drugs fairly often, but they no longer were violent or angry.

This was a pivotal moment in my life. By approaching a frightening and potentially devastating aspect of my career with a courage and willingness to learn, I was able to empower myself and change my whole experience.

More Than Just a Mindset

Attitude is more than just a positive mindset. It affects how you think and behave, the activities you take part in, the choices you make—truly every part of your life! It's a pretty huge umbrella, and even though attitude is aligned with five of the 7 Keys: love, lifestyle, emotions, patience and persistence, and trusting the process, it fits most precisely into the 3rd Key because there is something specifically decisive and active about your attitude. It doesn't just happen; you have to make a choice and work on it consistently.

The question is, how do you shift your attitude when you feel stuck? If you're going through something difficult, like the healing process, it can be really challenging to keep your perspective positive and lean into your growth. It's normal to feel that it's never going to get better, that it's never going to end. The practice is to focus on *believing* that your situation can change. Changing your attitude is a lot about trusting and moving forward.

Obviously, love helps! If you approach your life, make decisions and take actions from your heart, the impact will be more lasting and beneficial. For example, rather than saying "I *have to* quit smoking," instead you can say, "I want to be my healthiest self. I love my body, so I will no longer smoke." If you deny yourself something out of a feeling of obligation or guilt, you may be perpetuating the feelings that made you want to do that thing in the first place. You won't stop feeling deprived by depriving yourself.

The other reason that attitude is so linked to the 3rd Key is that lifestyle choices can improve your attitude. Exercise, diet, and sleep all have a direct correlation to how you feel and interface with the world. If you feel discouraged, go for a hike in the woods. Go for a swim. Go to bed early and sleep in. You might be surprised how your perspective can change just through these simple steps.

Actions and Exercises for the 6th Fundamental Attitude

1. **Practice Gratitude**

   Science shows that gratitude is the best way to generate positivity. When you have a practice of being grateful for your life, it helps change your attitude and move you toward positivity.

2. **Do an Attitude Adjustment**

   If you have a situation in your life that is bothering you, but you feel helpless to change it, you may begin to feel frustrated. It may be the hours you work, or how much you have to drive your kids around, or when your husband comes home from work. A lot of times, these situations are marked by our feeling of not being in control of that event. An attitude adjustment takes you to a different place, one where you can feel in control of what you are doing. It can be as simple as recognizing that you agreed to work for this company that gave you the hours you work. Or that you want your children to be good at something, so that's why you're driving them around.

For example, when I was going to acupuncture school, I was also working in the ER, so I always got the night shifts and weekends, which no one else wanted. Initially my attitude was one of anger that I didn't get better shifts. But then I did an attitude adjustment, and I realized that I wanted to be in acupuncture school, so my availability for the job was the hours I was being given, and at least I had a good job!

3. **Walk a Mile**

   We all have particular ideas about people or places we've been. We can't help it; it's a natural part of our existence. Often in our everyday lives there may be a person or group of people who provoke us to feel a certain way, or upset us for some reason. I use an exercise called "walking a mile" in someone else's shoes to help me be more understanding toward that person. There are several ways to do this.
   - You can ask the person why they behave in a way that provokes you. Most people have a reason for what they're doing: all you have to do is be curious enough to ask them what's going on. They will probably tell you, with great clarity.
   - You can try to understand their history: what might be contributing to their behavior? Perhaps a woman was abused by her parents, which made her feel really insecure, or a man who grew up in another country might have different customs, which make him behave in a way that doesn't make sense to you.

~ Chapter 4

4th Key: Listening to Your Body

"There is more wisdom in your body than in your deepest philosophies."
—FRIEDRICH NIETZSCHE

COMMUNICATION IS VITAL

"Symptoms are in fact merely a special type of body language."
—RUEDIGER DAHLKE

Everything you feel physically is a communication. When you have a stomachache, when you feel tired, when your head hurts, when your body aches—these are all different ways that your body tells you to pay attention. Sometimes when your body speaks it's totally obvious what's going on, but other times the signs are more subtle.

Have you ever had the experience of not knowing that your back is sore until you receive a massage? Or not realizing that you were hungry until you sat down to eat? We are all busy, and stressed, and going about our lives not noticing how a particular food is affecting our energy, or how a specific exercise is aggravating our back, or even how caffeine is affecting us. In order to take the steps necessary to heal your body, you first have to learn to understand what your body is trying to communicate.

It seems like listening to your body should be as intrinsic as breathing, but for most of us, it's more like learning a foreign language. I often talk about treating your body the way you would treat a pet. If your dog is whimpering, you try to figure out why. You don't ignore it, or say, "Shut up" or "Get over it!"

You empathize. You worry about what's wrong with it. You try to comfort it, take it to the vet, and do everything you can to make it feel better. Similarly, when your body is talking, you may not always understand the language, but you know that it is talking to you.

My body has always been very sensitive. I grew up with a perpetually stuffy nose, a symptom that lasted well into adulthood. Over the years, and as an adult, I tried many different things to make it better: acupuncture, craniosacral work, and I even had surgery to correct my deviated septum. Nothing helped.

Finally, I had a food allergy test and found that I was extremely allergic to dairy. It took me years to recognize my allergy because, like so many of us, I didn't want to give up certain foods. Even though on some level I knew dairy was a problem for me, I loved my cheese, my ice cream, and in the winter, my eggnog latte.

After finding out that my reactivity to dairy was off the charts, I looked back and realized that my dairy allergy had been there since birth. As a baby, I had to be taken off formula because I kept getting sick. I remember being forced to drink milk at the dinner table as a child and hating it.

Once I stopped eating dairy, my nose cleared up completely! It was a long journey to learn that dairy was my problem, and my body had been trying to tell me the whole time!

In life, *you* are the one having the experience. You have the capacity to become an expert in what feels good in your own body and to understand the signals that your body expresses, and you do not have to have medical expertise to be able to do this. You do need the willingness and desire to listen, take action and be consistent about it, especially when your body is speaking to you.

LISTENING TO HEAL

My new patients often complain on their first visit that they are not healing in the way they want to heal. We tend to have fixed perceptions of what our healing is going to look like, but when the prescribed and obvious remedy doesn't work, *there's something else that needs to be addressed.* If the condition is particularly obstinate, chronic, or mysterious, usually that *"something else"* is rather difficult to see or hear.

The question is, why it is so difficult to hear your own body?

For one thing, we live in a very loud world. We are inundated with so many stimuli in our day-to-day lives that our ability to process our experiences is affected. We build certain coping mechanisms just to be able to be in the world, and have essentially become desensitized to listening because of all the noise around us.

A lot of times, ignoring the sensitivities in our bodies seems easier than trying to explore what's going on. As long as we're not in pain or struggling with some issue, our health is just one less thing to worry about. If your stomach is just *a little* upset after eating pasta carbonara, and it's one of your favorite foods, why worry?

Listening to your body can feel overwhelming. Where do you begin? It can feel like opening a can of worms, and you may feel you don't have time to deal with everything that's going to come up. Or maybe you fear that you won't be able to hear your body, or maybe there are things you don't want to hear. Like me, you may not *want* to know that you're allergic to dairy, or that you're going to have to change your lifestyle in order to give your body what it needs.

As you learn to listen to your body, you'll most likely become more sensitive. At the same time, you develop a strength inside that allows you to feel more tolerant of what you are experiencing, with less need to protect yourself.

Listening to your body is a choice you make all the time. It is one of the most empowering elements of your own healing, because it allows you to take charge and not feel so frightened and hopeless. Your body becomes a mirror, allowing you to see yourself more clearly, move forward and grow into the life that you desire.

Fundamentals of the 4th Key
Listening to Your Body

The 4th Key, Listening to Your Body, is deeply woven into each of the 7 Keys, and resides in the center of the 7 Keys. Having strengthened your commitment and the stability in your body through the first three keys, you are now ready to be able to listen to the deeper messages in your body and move forward into the final three keys with greater authority and vision.

Much of this chapter focuses on your symptoms, since they are the gateway for you to be able to learn more about what your body needs and how to feel better. The 4th Key helps you learn to be more attuned to both instinct and logic, and to distinguish fear from truth.

1st Fundamental: Observation

Do you know when you're hungry? When you are sleepy? When you don't feel well? The first step to listening to your body is to take stock of what you already know. Learning *how* to observe and *how* to listen are tremendous tools throughout the healing process.

4th Key: Listening to Your Body

2nd Fundamental: What's Wrong?
Taking an inventory and understanding your symptoms is a crucial step to healing. You can't really know how to fix something unless you know what's wrong. It's important to pay attention to all the different aspects of your health, and not just focus on the one thing bothering you the most. In this way, you can have a more holistic and long-term approach to your health and healing.

3rd Fundamental: Symptoms and the Organ Systems
According to Chinese medicine, your symptoms are clear indicators of where your body is out of balance. By learning which symptoms relate to which organs, you can take that information and apply it to your healing process—through exercises, supplements, diet, and working with healers to bring your body into equilibrium.

4th Fundamental: Listening and the Emotions
Emotions by their nature can cloud our thinking. When we're afraid of something, or holding on to anger about something, it will block our ability to feel what is happening in our bodies. One of the main elements of getting well when it seems impossible is understanding that emotions play a huge role in our health. But they also play a huge role in blocking us from feeling our bodies, which is what we are addressing here.

1st Fundamental
Observation

START WITH THE URGENT SITUATIONS

In order to be able to hear and understand your own body, you first need to address any immediate and dangerous problems. Pain is a loud signal from your body telling you to do something different right away. If you sprained your ankle, the pain and swelling tells you to stay off it, to let it heal. If you move the wrong way, a sudden sharp pain will signal you to "STOP." This is how your body talks to you, and one way that you already know how to listen.

If your symptoms are acute, or if pain is affecting your mobility, your work, or your sense of well-being, don't wait; get help right away. You won't be able to hear anything else in your body when all of your attention is focused on your pain. The 2nd Key gave you tools to create a stable foundation by balancing your digestion, hormones, immune system, and nervous system, but if you are still in pain, start with the urgent situations. Part of listening to your body is knowing when to seek immediate help.

THE POWER OF OBSERVATION

Once you have determined that you are not in immediate danger, begin to observe the sensations in your body. This may be the first time you really begin paying attention to your body. We all notice the basic survival signals such as hunger, thirst, sleepiness, or pain, but we actually know so much more about our body's wants and needs.

For example, when you go out to lunch, how do you decide what to eat? You might want salad, or soup, or something more meaty and substantial. Whether you know it or not, your body is telling you what it wants to eat, and that becomes your decision. It should be noted: if you constantly want to eat macaroni and cheese and ice cream for lunch, this is not likely a message

4th Key: Listening to Your Body

about the nutrients your body needs, but you can still pay attention to it. If you have cravings that you know are bad for you, it doesn't mean you should act on them, but you can still observe them and try to understand what's going on internally.

There are countless ways your body speaks to you every day. We all have gut reactions or instincts we can't explain. When you walk into a room and get butterflies, your body is telling you something—to be alert and pay attention. When we feel exhausted for no apparent reason, our body is begging for rest, nourishment, and support. Even our cravings and addictions can help us learn what our body really needs.

In order to understand what your body is saying and make the changes needed for it to heal, it takes commitment to the relationship. You want to show up for your body every day. Every time you eat, every time you exercise, pay attention. Listen. You may have moments where you choose to eat something you know your body doesn't love, but do it consciously. Choose to eat that cinnamon roll, and love it in totality if that's what you are choosing. And then pay attention to how it affects you. Just because you're doing something you think may be "unhealthy," doesn't mean that you should stop paying attention.

Initially, when you begin observing, don't change anything (unless, of course, you are in crisis and you need to address it immediately). If you can, simply observe. You've already worked to clear the noise from your body through the 3rd Key, so you are already more sensitive to hear it. Acquaint yourself with your habits, body, moods, and energy levels. This simple practice will allow you to see what works and what doesn't work in your health and lifestyle. Eventually, you'll learn to hear the more subtle signals in your body.

BEING A GOOD LISTENER

Consider your family and friends. Who is a good listener, and what are the qualities that make you want to confide in someone? What makes you feel heard?

Good listeners don't make assumptions or think they already know the answer. They ask questions, really pay attention when you answer, and then ask follow-up questions to gain clarity. They aren't thinking about how they are going to respond, or concerned with their own agenda. They are completely present, undistracted, and focused on you. They help you understand yourself better, simply by reflecting their experience of what you are saying.

Can you bring these qualities to listening to your own body? Can you simply ask your body questions without judgement or agenda?

Actions for the 1st Fundamental Observation

1. **Observe Your Hunger**

    Make a practice of observing your hunger. Ask yourself these questions:
    - When does your body signal that it's hungry? Is it the same time every day? If it's different, did anything different occur in your life that may have affected your hunger level (i.e. Did you wake up earlier? Did you work out harder? Was it a warm day or a hot day? Etc).
    - Are you able to stop and eat when you are hungry, or do you only eat at the appointed times?
    - How do you feel before you eat? How is your mood? How do you feel after you eat?
    - Are you craving certain foods?

- Do you know what your body likes to eat?
- What foods fill you up quickly? Do you get hungry again shortly after?
- Are there other any observations you notice about your hunger?

2. Observe Your Sleep

When does your body tell you it is sleepy?
- Are you most energetic in the morning or in the evening?
- Do you get the afternoon doldrums?
- How do you feel after a good night's sleep, or after a poor night's sleep?
- Do you feel that you sleep enough? Does the alarm always wake you? Do you have to drag yourself out of bed?

It would be best to do this exercise for a week, but at a minimum, three days will give you an indication. Write down what you notice in a journal or notebook. Writing things down helps you slow down and truly observe your experiences. Pay attention to one thing at a time so you don't get overwhelmed. Keeping a journal also allows you to look back at your observations. You may be surprised by what you learn.

2nd Fundamental
What's Wrong?

RON

My patient Ron had moved across the country, but he called me one day because he wasn't feeling well. At first he just felt a little ill, but then he was constipated for eight days. He called me every day to discuss his symptoms. Obviously, he was concerned and frightened (because he was calling me every day), but he seemed blocked by his fear and somehow unable to really tune in to be able to express to me what he was feeling. He couldn't really describe specific symptoms, he said he just felt "wrong."

Early on, I had the idea that he had appendicitis, but he said there was no specific pain in that area of his body and he really didn't want to go to the ER. Eventually he started to have a fever and I told him to go to the emergency room. It turned out his appendix had ruptured! After emergency surgery and a month on antibiotics, he felt better.

How long have you lived with your symptoms? People often live with symptoms for years, as long as they're not life threatening. In order to be healthy, you have to pay attention to the places in your body that aren't feeling good, which means focusing on your symptoms. As you explore the signals your body is sending, you learn what is going to work for you and what isn't. By following the pain in your body, you can use the source of your pain as the point of change.

Begin to observe your symptoms. Having already done a cleanse and studied your hunger and sleep, you'll notice more about the symptoms in your body. *What doesn't feel right? How was it when it felt well?* Some people live with symptoms all day and think it's OK—such as heartburn, or a stuffy nose. Try to pay attention, without emotion, judgment or fear. What is the pain in your body trying to tell you?

4th Key: Listening to Your Body

It can be overwhelming to listen to your body if you're experiencing a lot of symptoms or pain. If that's the case, start with whatever is bothering you the most. Start with one symptom and explore it. Everything is probably connected, so if you attend to one symptom, the others will also likely be affected.

You can learn so much about yourself and your body through your symptoms. For example, if your stomach is upset, you will learn in this chapter and in the next chapter on emotions that the stomach is connected to the emotion of worry. It could help you to eat warm, cooked foods, since they are easier to digest, and if you can find ways to reduce your worry and stress, your digestion may improve.

With Chinese medicine as a framework, you can discover what may be behind your symptoms and begin to take the steps to heal.

THE ENERGY TIMELINE

In Chinese medicine, there is an energy timeline that a physical issue follows before it becomes visible and impossible to ignore. It moves something like this:

1. Your Qi falls out of balance and harmony due to stress, diet, lifestyle changes, environmental factors, emotions, etc.
2. Your internal organs begin to show signs of energetic dysfunction (which can be ascertained by Chinese medicine diagnostic methods). Organs begin to develop problems communicating with other organs.
3. The issue becomes a physical problem. This is the point at which Western medicine tests can diagnose with relative accuracy.

Your body may be speaking to you long before symptoms become acute, or even before they are diagnosable through standard medical tests. A single physiological imbalance can turn into a cascade of imbalances and ailments by the time we seek help. By that time, it can be a challenge to know where and what to begin treating first

In the process of learning to listen to your body, you may be able to hear the more subtle signals—things that show up earlier on the energy timeline—so that you can take the needed steps to bring yourself back to balance before an issue fully develops. Sometimes, though, a problem may be so deep that the solution is not immediately obvious. It may take time for results to be revealed.

As you learn to listen to your body, you'll begin to understand when you need to take action, and when you need to practice patience with the process.

THE SPIRITUAL AND EMOTIONAL ASPECT OF SYMPTOMS

Rudiger Dahlke is a medical doctor and psychotherapist who examines the connection between the body, mind, and spirit. He believes that all physical issues are at root spiritual issues that our soul is asking us to address. In his essay, "Disease as the Language of the Soul," he states: *"The following questions have been shown to be helpful when making a diagnosis: Why is this happening to me at this time? What does the symptom stop me from doing? What does it force me to do? What sense does it have in my life at this time?"* (Dahlke, Disease as the Language of the Soul, 1979)

If you are experiencing pain, how might your emotions play a part? Did something happen in your life that precipitated the symptoms? While we will be exploring the results of these questions further in the next few chapters, it is helpful to begin to assess your symptoms and the connection they have to your emotions, since *your symptoms are more than just physical.*

4th Key: Listening to Your Body

Actions and Exercises for the 2nd Fundamental What's Wrong?

1. **Take an inventory of all your symptoms:** Go through your entire body, from your head to your feet.
    - Am I holding tension in my body? Where am I holding on? If I breathe into that place, will it loosen up?
    - Is my body aching? What aches? How does it ache?
    - Am I tired? If I sleep, will I feel better, or is it a deeper tiredness?
    - Do I have a headache?
    - Am I congested in my lungs or in my sinuses?
    - How is my digestion?
    - Am I feeling emotional? What emotions?
    - Am I stressed? How do I know when I feel stressed?
    - And so on ...

2. **Take a deeper exploration of your symptoms. For each symptom, ask yourself:**
    - When did it start?
    - How bad is it—on a scale of 1-10?
    - How often does it happen?
    - What makes it better?
    - What makes it worse?

If you don't know what makes it better and what makes it worse, try taking action so you can begin to understand what might help or hinder the pain. For example, is it worse at night or during the day? Or all the time? Does it get worse when you walk? Or when you sit for a long time? Or when

Healing When It Seems Impossible

you dance? When you eat a certain food, does it make you feel sick? Do you have trouble breathing? These are all important observations.

3. **Gain awareness in your body.** If you have recurring pain in your body, the next time your body hurts, don't take a painkiller, don't get angry, don't do whatever it is that you would normally do. Instead:
    - Describe the pain: is it sharp, is it dull, is it radiating, is it throbbing ...?
    - Does it feel like it is connected to any other part of your body (*i.e.*, when your shoulder hurts, do you also feel it in your thumb, etc.)?
    - How do you feel emotionally? Are you upset, sad, angry, worried?
    - What were you thinking about immediately preceding the onset of the pain?
    - If you woke up with the pain, what were you thinking/experiencing when you went to sleep, or did you have any odd dreams?
    - Are there any recent changes in your diet, exercise, physical reality (did you recently change jobs, change homes, etc)?

You can also do this in relation to other physical symptoms like nausea, cramping, etc.

4. **Explore where emotions might be stuck in your body.** The location of where you experience emotional pain in your body, or where the physical pain is, can help indicate what might need attention.
    - When you feel emotional, pay attention to how your body feels. Write down where the emotions are showing up in your body. For example, if you are feeling pain in your chest, it may be your lungs, which are related to grief in Chinese medicine. Is there something you feel you've lost?

4th Key: Listening to Your Body

- In a journal, write down where you physically feel pain, and describe any emotions or memories that come up in connection to the pain.

3rd Fundamental
Symptoms and the Organ Systems

MARY

Mary suddenly began to feel afraid of everything. She had no other symptoms. She came in to see me because she "knew" something was wrong. In Chinese medicine, fear is the emotion connected to kidneys, which also rule the lower back, knees, bones, energy levels, adrenal gland, and the physical brain. Because acupuncture and Chinese herbs alone didn't help her, I began to suspect there was something else going on. Testing revealed that she had a brain tumor, and because she listened to her body, she discovered it early enough to treat.

ORGAN SYSTEMS

In my practice, I work to uncover the root of a problem in order to create healing. Rather than chasing symptoms, I pull at the threads of symptoms and unravel the underlying problem. Even if the symptoms appear very different, they usually end up being interconnected.

Even without the vigorous training of Chinese medicine schooling, you can use Chinese medicine as a framework to better understand the language of your own body. Obviously, there is so much more involved than what I am able to describe here. I have been studying and practicing Chinese medicine for more than 25 years … and I'm still learning!

The information I have included here is meant to be a springboard for you to be able to understand your body better, and to play with what might make it feel more nourished, supported, and strong.

To understand this further, we need to look at the organ systems and the meridians in your body. The practice of Chinese medicine focuses on 12 major organs. Each organ has a meridian, or a pathway of energy, that is connected to the organ and the particular functions of that organ. These meridians are where *Qi* (life force energy) flows. The energy extends from each organ, along its energetic pathway through the body, and ends at the fingers and toes. Acupuncture is one tool that helps balance the movement of energy in the body so it can heal itself naturally. *(*You can read more about acupuncture and the organ systems in **Appendix A–Chinese medicine 101***)*.

Furthermore, each organ has different and additional functions in Chinese medicine. For example, the spleen makes blood, but in Chinese medicine the spleen also regulates the strength of muscles, transports the energy of food, affects your ability to concentrate, and is ruled by the emotion of worry. This is just one example, and a few of the functions that Chinese medicine attributes to a particular organ. Each organ has emotional and spiritual functions, sensory functions (the liver regulates the eyes, the kidneys regulate the ears, etc.), a time of the day that it is functioning optimally, a season, an element (the lungs relate to metal, the heart to fire, etc.), a flavor, and much, much more associated with it. There also are specific ways each organ interacts and relates to the other organs. These attributes are covered in more detail in following chapter about the emotions (**Chapter 5, 2nd Fundamental**) and in **Appendix A—Chinese medicine 101.**

When an organ is out of balance, you have symptoms that correspond to its functions. So, if you are experiencing sore muscles, nausea, low energy, and a feeling of anxiousness, you may have a spleen imbalance.

Or, if your symptoms are worse at a particular time of day, it may be linked to an organ's most active time of day. A common example of this is when you are tired in the late afternoon, which is the time of the kidney, so your kidneys may be out of balance. If you regularly wake up in the night at

4th Key: Listening to Your Body

1 am, that is the time of the liver, so your liver may be out of balance. You can use the Organ Time Clock in **Appendix A—Chinese medicine 101** as a reference.

With basic understanding of the functions of your organs, you can begin to interpret what is happening in your body. All of my patients who have been working with me for any length of time have learned to read their own bodies and know which organ is bothering them when they have symptoms, and what to do about it.

Learning to understand your body with Chinese medicine principles is like looking up into the night sky with knowledge of the constellations. Rather than seeing a multitude of individual stars (or symptoms), you can begin to understand the connections between them, and navigate your way more clearly using Chinese medicine as your guide.

YIN AND YANG ORGANS

Below is a list of symptoms connected to each of the organ systems. As you will notice, each organ is Yin or Yang in essence and has a corresponding partner organ. For example, the spleen (Yin), is partner to the stomach (Yang). Their functions are connected, and they work together to keep the body in balance. Their symptoms are also related to each other and have been grouped as such.

Yin organs produce, transform, regulate and store the body's fluids, blood, and Qi, while Yang organs are mainly responsible for digesting food and transmitting nutrients in the body. Yin organs play a more important role in Chinese medicine, but both are necessary to maintain and stabilize balance in the body.

A Map Towards Healing

Using the list of symptoms you inventoried in the 2nd Fundamental, you can begin to explore which organs may be out of balance and require support and attention. This is a huge step in learning to listen to your body. With this information, your symptoms become a map toward your healing.

It is important to keep in mind that just because you are experiencing symptoms that relate to a particular organ, doesn't mean you are "sick." If you are experiencing lower back pain, knee pain, fatigue, and a ringing in your ears, it does not mean your kidneys are failing, or that you have kidney cancer—it may just be an imbalance that needs attention. By understanding which organ is out of balance, you can respond to the messages your body is sending you and make the changes needed to heal. This includes dietary changes, supplements, exercises, and emotional and spiritual exploration and release. Of course, it would be great to work with a practitioner who can further help you understand and move toward solving the mysteries in your body.

There are specific actions for each organ system listed below. You will also find additional exercises that support the functioning of specific organs in the next chapter on Emotions.

As I've said before, be aware of any danger signs when you are listening to your body. Certain things should be taken care of immediately, so you want to make sure your symptoms are not life threatening, or something that requires you to go to the emergency room. You can find a list of 911 symptoms in **Appendix B**. Once you have ascertained that you are not in immediate danger, you can begin the process of investigation and listening to understand your body.

4th Key: Listening to Your Body

SYMPTOMS AND THE ORGAN SYSTEMS

HEART (Yin)—Small Intestines (Yang)

The HEART is considered the emperor of the internal organs and encompasses the emotional, spiritual, and mental aspects of all other organs. It houses the spiritual aspect of the mind, called the "Shen." The heart is responsible for good sleep, mental activity, consciousness, and thinking. The heart pathway ends at the tongue and rules the sense of taste, so the appearance of the tongue commonly reflects what is happening in the heart. It rules the emotion of joy. The element is fire, the season is Summer, and the flavor is bitter.

The SMALL INTESTINES are the Yang organ for the heart. Their job is to separate the clear from the turbid. When food is broken down in the small intestines, some components are absorbed through the intestinal lining and others are sent through to the large intestines as waste. The small intestines also do this with thought processes: when your thinking is unclear, it is connected to an imbalance in the small intestines.

Specific Symptoms related to the Heart and Small Intestine

- Tongue (problems with speech, talking incessantly, speaking rapidly, stuttering)
- Heart Attack
- Chest pain
- Heart palpitations, arrhythmias
- Mania, craziness, can't stop talking, laughing inappropriately
- Red complexion
- Not being able to sleep, insomnia
- Bitter taste in the mouth
- Blood vessels (varicose veins)
- Inability to think clearly

ACTIONS FOR STRENGTHENING THE HEART

The heart meridian starts in the armpit, extends down the inner part of the arm, and ends at the pinkie. Therefore, arm exercises can be particularly helpful to strengthen the heart. Try clenching your fists: sit up straight and allow your hands to rest comfortably between your thighs. Then, slowly make fists, exhaling while clenching, inhale while loosening. Do this 6 times.

> **Clean your teeth!** It has been recently shown that the physical heart can be damaged by gum disease and tooth problems.
>
> **Red:** The color associated with the heart is red, so red foods nourish the heart (like tomatoes, cherries, beets, apples and rhubarb).

LUNGS (Yin)—Large Intestines (Yang)

The LUNGS govern Qi (our "life force" or "life energy") and respiration. They are in charge of inhaling air and, as such, are the intermediary between the inside and the outside world. They are the main protector of the immune system. If lung function is healthy, skin and hair will have luster. The lung meridian ends at the nose, and rules the sense of smell. The emotion connected to the lungs is grief, the season is Fall, the flavor is spicy, and the element is metal.

The LARGE INTESTINES are the Yang organ of the lungs. Their job is to help the body get rid of waste, which is the same as its Western function. When your immune system is weak, the two things likely to show up first are diarrhea and upper respiratory infections.

Specific Symptoms related to the Lungs and Large Intestine

- Issues with sense of smell (nose)
- Respiration, shortness of breath
- Sinuses (sinus infection)
- Congestion
- Sore throat
- Voice (losing your voice)
- Cough
- Asthma
- Diarrhea
- Constipation
- Skin problems (acne, rashes, etc.)
- Getting sick a lot (immune system problems)
- Thyroid problems (connected to immune system)
- Gas and bloating (large intestines)
- Grief (sadness, depression, repressed emotions)

ACTIONS FOR THE LUNGS: DEEP BREATHING

Breathe in deeply through your nose. Fill your lungs and belly as you count to five. Then, hold your breath for a count of five. Exhale all of your air slowly through your nose, again counting to five. Once fully empty, hold again briefly before you begin the process again. You can do this process five times, or set a timer and do it for two minutes or longer. Try to do this at least once a day and note the effects!

White: The color associated with the lungs is white, so foods like white meat, tofu, radish, and mushrooms can benefit the lungs.

SPLEEN (YIN)—STOMACH (YANG)

The main function of the SPLEEN is to assist the stomach with digestion by transporting and transforming food essences, absorbing the nourishment from food and separating out the usable aspect of food. It controls the blood by making sure it stays in the vessels, controls the strength of the muscles, the movement of the limbs, and ends in the mouth/lips. The spleen rules our ability to focus and concentrate and the emotion of worry. Its spiritual function has to do with being able to receive. The season is late Summer, the element is Earth, and the flavor is sweet. People crave sweets when the spleen is out of balance.

The STOMACH is the Yang organ paired with the spleen and controls the cooking of food; it prepares food to be digested. Its job is to *send energy down* and transport food essence through the digestive tract to continue the process of digestion. (Every organ has a direction of energy, and the stomach's direction is downward. If it moves upward, it comes up as a burp or vomit.) It is also the origin of fluids, in that it extracts fluids from the food you eat to be used by the body and then filtered by the kidneys.

Specific Symptoms related to the Spleen and Stomach

- Heartburn
- Stomachaches - Indigestion
- Nausea, vomiting
- Diarrhea
- Stomach distension
- Craving sweets
- Difficulty waking in the morning
- Varicose veins
- Rebellious Qi: burping, vomiting (stomach Qi in wrong direction)
- Feeling full quickly (loss of appetite)
- Worry (anxiety, obsessive worrying)
- Inability to concentrate
- Muscle aches
- Fatigue
- Bad breath
- Easy bruising
- Weakness or heaviness in limbs
- Pale complexion
- Bleeding without being able to stop (heavy periods)
- The spiritual function has to do with receiving

4th Key: Listening to Your Body

Actions for the Spleen: Chew Your food!

One thing that you can do immediately to help your spleen and stomach is to chew your food well. Chew it slowly, and don't be distracted while you're eating. Make your food a pleasurable meditation, and see what happens to you emotionally.

Yellow: The color associated with the spleen is yellow, so yellow foods (including bananas, squash, peppers, oats, beans) can all benefit the spleen.

LIVER (Yin)—Gallbladder (Yang)

The LIVER is like a military commander in the body, responsible for overall planning of the body's functions and ensuring a smooth flow of energy throughout the whole body. Because of this, the liver can override other organs, so when the energy is not moving properly, it can affect the symptoms of other organs. The liver also influences our ability to see the big picture and have a sense of direction in life. It is the source of courage and resoluteness. It stores the blood, regulates the menstrual flow, and controls the sinews. Most menstrual problems such as PMS, cramps, and migraines are connected to liver imbalances. It regulates emotions, digestion and secretion of bile. The emotion is anger, the element is wood, the season is Spring, and the flavor is sour.

The GALLBLADDER is the Yang organ paired with the liver. It stores and secretes bile, it regulates the ligaments and tendons, and it rules the ability to make decisions. When you are trying to get too much done or under extreme stress, the gallbladder is the organ that acts up. This includes getting actual gallbladder pain, side aches, headaches, neck aches, or even sciatica, but also includes difficulty making decisions or moving forward in your plans.

Specific Symptoms related to the Liver and Gallbladder

- Eye issues (dry or bloodshot eyes, floaters, blurry vision, poor night vision, styes)
- Shoulder and neck (neck ache, shoulder ache, feeling of a lump in your throat)
- Ligaments and tendons (sprains, strains)
- Menstrual cycle issues (PMS, cramps, fibroids, endometriosis)
- a feeling of a lump in your throat
- Irritability or outbursts of anger, frustration
- Depression, repressed anger
- Prostate issues
- Migraines and headaches
- High blood pressure
- Stroke
- Gallbladder and liver problems
- Indecisiveness
- Sciatica
- Extreme stress
- Side aches
- Influences our ability to see the big picture and have a sense of direction in life.
- The source of courage and resoluteness
- Alcohol addiction

ACTIONS FOR THE LIVER: ACUPRESSURE FOR THE LIVER!

There is an acupressure point that you can massage to unblock the liver Qi. The spot is right between the big toe bone and the second toe bone on both feet. Using your thumb, or the heel of your other foot, massage this point on both feet every day. If it is sore, that means it is blocked, and you are hitting the right spot!

Green: The color associated with the liver is green, so eat your green vegetables to maintain liver health!

KIDNEYS (Yin)—Urinary Bladder (Yang)

The KIDNEYS are the core of all life force energy. They determine the basic constitution, strength, and vitality of all other organs. They control the energy of important life transitions such as birth, puberty, menopause, and death. Aging itself is due to decline in kidney energy. Kidneys produce the matrix of the bones, bone marrow, spinal cord, and brain. They control the lower back, knees, and overall energy level. They also control the flow of water in the body. The kidneys regulate your hearing and your ears. Fear is the emotion associated with kidney function. They also house your willpower. Salt is the flavor, water is the element, and Winter is the season associated with the kidneys.

The URINARY BLADDER is the Yang organ that is paired with the kidneys. The bladder carries out the physiological functions of the kidneys. It handles the metabolism of water, affects dreams, and supports the kidneys.

Specific Symptoms related to the Kidneys and Urinary Bladder

- Urinary pain
- Fear
- Lower back pain
- Knee pain
- Fatigue (severe fatigue)
- Memory Loss
- Head injuries
- Hearing problems
- Tinnitus (also liver)
- Physical matter of the brain
- Depression in the classic sense —low serotonin
- Bones
- Overall sense of having energy
- Menopausal symptoms
- Big transitions in life
- "Salt" addiction

ACTIONS FOR THE KIDNEYS: RUB YOUR KIDNEYS

In order to support your kidneys, or help if you are feeling fear, rub your kidneys. Your kidneys are located on your back, below your lowest ribs (not your low back as many people think). Rub them in a circular motion 49 times. (Seven times seven is an auspicious number in Chinese culture.)

Black: The color associated with the kidneys is black, so eating black foods (like black beans, black rice, black lentils and blackberries) is beneficial for the kidneys.

COMPLEX ISSUES

There are several common conditions that are influenced by different organs, depending on the circumstances. If you suffer from one of these conditions, you can look at your other symptoms in order to understand which organ may be the one that is most affected. For example, if you are depressed, and you also have migraines, shoulder and neck pain, and menstrual issues, it is likely that your depression may be stemming from a liver imbalance. Below are a list of these conditions and the organs that are connected to them.

ALLERGIES

- **Liver:** Springtime allergies are connected to the liver. Doing a liver detox in the spring can make a huge difference. The liver is also sensitive to wind, which is common in springtime, and makes allergies worse.
- **Spleen:** If you have trouble digesting or absorbing your food, it can affect your immune system and thereby increase your allergy symptoms.

- **Lungs:** Allergies affect the immune system, so the symptoms often show up in the lung meridian, even if the origin is in the liver.

Pregnancy Issues

- **Liver:** The liver regulates menstrual cycles and helps support the smooth flow of energy in the whole body.
- **Spleen:** Weakness and anemia.
- **Lungs (immune system):** Deficient thyroid is related to immune system issues, and is a common problem for women who are having trouble getting pregnant. Recently, I had four patients with this problem who began taking thyroid medication, and they have all have since become pregnant!
- **Kidneys:** The kidneys rule your overall sense of having energy, which translates into your adrenal glands and sex hormones. If you have weak kidney energy, you may not have enough hormones to get pregnant or hold a pregnancy.

Depression

- **Spleen:** Excess worry.
- **Lungs:** Grief—holding onto grief.
- **Liver:** Anger. A lot of people who are depressed are angry underneath.
- **Heart:** Lack of joy.
- **Kidneys:** Fear. Also, the kidneys affect the brain chemistry and if brain chemistry is out of balance it affects depression.

Sleep Issues

The inability to sleep is not just one thing. Most commonly it is:
- **Liver:** Trouble with falling asleep
- **Heart or Lungs:** Trouble staying asleep
- **Heart or Liver:** Nightmares
- **Spleen:** Insomnia—can't stop worrying.

4th Fundamental
Listening and the Emotions

Listening Despite Fear

Emotions, by their nature, can cloud or distort our thinking. If you're exercising, you're so full of endorphins you might feel like you can push your body more than it's capable and end up pulling a muscle. When you are angry or upset, it can be difficult to think straight, let alone become quiet enough to hear the subtle signals your body is sending. It can be difficult to discern fear from intuition.

Emotions can make our internal experience so noisy that there is no space to hear the body. The 5th Key is dedicated to the emotional element of our health, but it is important to mention here, because our emotions can disrupt our ability to hear.

Learning to listen to your body requires both logic and intuition because there are emotional elements that arise when we listen to our bodies. Often, we interpret our emotions as our heart—we *feel things* as truth—but this is not always correct. For example, fear might be alerting us to a dangerous condition so we can protect ourselves, but fear is often imaginary and only serves to keep us from seeing what's really right for us. How do you discern between fear and fact? How do you get to that deeper place of listening?

4th Key: Listening to Your Body

When a person has a serious illness, finding the way to healing is like hiking a narrow path through a dense forest. Fear comes from all directions and threatens you in every way. The right answer is hard to feel. You can't be in a state of fear if you want to listen.

With a dangerous illness like cancer or HIV, there are often statistics that will predict the outcome. It is difficult not to buy into the prevailing medical opinion about that condition. Try to remember that no matter what statistics say, you are an individual. What is right for you may be unique to your body and needs. As a physician, I help people find the truth for themselves. I offer choices and give my opinion of which will work best for you, but in the end, the decision of which path to take through the forest is yours.

Many times someone's fear is heightened because they feel there isn't enough time to discover the right treatment. And as we know, the sensation of fear increases stressors in the body, making it even more challenging to listen to what is best for your body. Unless you're in the most acute circumstances, allow yourself the time to ask questions and find the answers you need. Ask your body: "What do you need? What should I do next?"

Take time to really reflect on what it is you want for your healing. How does it look and feel? Allow the inner knowing to come through so you can make a choice that makes sense. If chemotherapy, as an example, is the best option, decide that for yourself.

Twenty years ago, Marty was diagnosed with thyroid cancer. Radiation and surgery were prescribed as cures. One morning, he woke up and realized that he needed to sing. He refused conventional treatment and took opera lessons. Using his voice in a new way changed something inside him, and his cancer was healed. His decision to heal came from deep within, and he was able to listen to it without letting the fear take him over.

IRENE

Irene had been trying to get pregnant for four years. She and her husband had tried everything—in vitro fertilization, hormones, and so on. She told me "If one more person tells me to relax, and that it'll happen when I quit worrying, I'm going to scream!" She already blamed herself. She was angry with her body for not doing what she wanted it to do, and knowing that her stress might be the cause of her inability to become pregnant simply caused her more stress.

When Irene and her husband finally gave up, and decided to quit trying, she almost immediately became pregnant. But her relaxation had to happen in its own time. Having people remind her not to worry, or blaming herself, did not help the situation. Sometimes life has its own agenda—its own divine timing.

RESPONSIBILITY WITHOUT BLAME

A common and dangerous pitfall of this healing process is blaming yourself (or others) for your condition. We want to understand "why" because it seems like that will lead to the solution—but why often just turns us in circles.

Taking responsibility for your health and healing is very different from taking responsibility for a mistake you've made. Imagine that your body is a business, and you are the business owner. If you mismanage it, of course there are consequences. But even if you are impeccable in every arena, you can't control the market—you can't control everything. There are things that are beyond our control, and our job is to figure out how to best deal with all the elements of our life and find our way to healing.

There is a subtle line between *feeling responsible and feeling culpable*. Feeling responsible means actively using your mind to focus on growth, solutions, and possibility. It is a daily, even a moment-by-moment practice. Rather than asking *"What did I do to deserve this?"* or *"Why is this happening to me?"* you can lighten your load by asking "What is my body trying to tell me? How can I listen and support my body and my healing?"

4th Key: Listening to Your Body

Remember: Healing is your goal and your body is on your side. When you remember this, everything takes on a different hue, including the illness itself.

Actions and Exercises for the 4th Fundamental Listening and the Emotions

Muscle Testing

You can ask your body anything and it will respond. You may have heard of "muscle testing," which is a method of diagnosing whether certain products or foods or nutritional supplements—or anything, really—is good for *your* body. It's really easy to muscle test yourself.

The easiest way is to hold something up to your chest. Try it with a packet of artificial sugar (since artificial sugar is universally bad). You will fall forward if it is good for you, or fall backward if it is bad for you. If you don't fall at all, it means that it is neutral. It's like a Ouija board for your body. Try it! (It helps sometimes to take a deep breath and relax as you are doing this.)

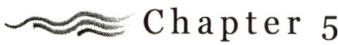# Chapter 5

5th Key: Emotions and Your Body

"The best and most beautiful things in the world cannot be seen or even touched. They must be felt with the heart."
—Helen Keller

"Let's not forget that the little emotions are the great captains of our lives and we obey them without realizing it."
—Vincent Van Gogh

JILL

Jill has been my patient for years. She is 52, and originally came to see me for help with symptoms of menopause. Recently, Jill started having heart palpitations. She went to a cardiologist and they found that she had an arrhythmia—an irregular heartbeat.

This information really scared Jill. She started to have trouble breathing and felt a heavy sensation in her chest. Her cardiologist wanted to give her a drug, but I told her that there was no reason she should have those new symptoms based upon her diagnosis of an irregularity of heartbeats.

I talked to Jill about the possibility that there was something emotional connected to her symptoms. She became quite angry. She said, "It's easy for you to say that it's emotional, but it's not my fault! You need to help me! I'm doing

5th Key: Emotions and Your Body

everything right! I lived my life doing what I thought was the right thing for me—so what could be going on?"

The truth is, Jill is an excellent patient and pretty much has everything going for her. She eats well and exercises regularly, cycling 25-50 miles on the weekends. She feels inspired by her career and is in love with her husband. She even spent time in therapy and has worked out many personal issues.

Her father was incredibly successful professionally, but he did not spend very much time with his family. When he died, he told her not to live her life like he did. Partly because of this, Jill has devoted her life to making the "right" choices and to living a balanced life. The idea that there could be something unseen causing her symptoms was especially devastating to her, because she had always been so focused on being healthy in every way.

I told her that her body could be expressing an emotional trauma that she might not remember. I told her that whatever was happening was not something that she was aware of, otherwise it would not be affecting her heart and her health. Most importantly, I told her that it was not about blaming her body or thinking she was somehow at fault; it was simply something to consider.

Jill then started to tell me that when she was a child she had heart problems. As she spoke, she began to relax. She told me that one of her siblings had died when she was young, and afterward she had felt that there was no room for her in the family. There was no nurturing around the loss of her sibling. We talked for a long while, and by the end of our time together Jill realized that some of the pressure in her chest was relieved.

She is continuing her journey, listening to her body, and finding tools to help her look into the story behind her symptoms. She started journaling, is seeing a therapist, and is continuing to have acupuncture. Jill can now see that her condition is not the result of doing something "wrong," but rather an opportunity for her to learn more about herself. She is looking at her experiences with curiosity, and trying to understand the possible emotional truths that are in her body and waiting to be revealed.

EMOTIONS ARE REAL

Generally, when we think about health we think about our body. The body is physical, functional, scientific, solid, and "real." Because it's "real," we feel we should be able to work with it in a purely physical and scientific fashion. From this perspective, it doesn't seem logical that our emotions and energy—which are not physical and more difficult to control—should influence the workings of our body. Yet, in life, we all know that our emotions affect our bodies.

Emotions almost always involve a physiological response. When we become angry, our face heats up and our blood races. When we are sad, our heart hurts and our throat constricts. When we are happy, our body feels light and stimulated. These are actual physical experiences of emotions, which means that we cannot separate our bodies from our emotions. Whether we hold them back or express them with fervor, emotions affect our bodies. They affect how we *feel* physically, and these feelings are quite *real*.

In my many years of practice, I have found that when someone has physical pain or symptoms that are not responding to treatment or appear to have an elusive diagnosis (*i.e.*, the source of the problem cannot be located through tests), *the answer will be found in the emotions.*

THE POWER OF EMOTIONS

Our emotions can be frightening. Our behavior changes when we experience heightened emotions, and we feel we have less control. Emotions blur our clarity and affect our decision-making abilities. Very often we don't even understand why we are experiencing certain emotions, or reacting in certain ways. It's no wonder that we squirm at the idea that our emotions affect our body and our health.

Like my patient Jill, many of us bristle at the idea that there is an emotional or spiritual component to an illness. We take it personally, or defensively—as if we are trying to get sick, or that we've done something wrong. Almost au-

5th Key: Emotions and Your Body

tomatically, we blame ourselves: *"If I am sick, and my emotions are part of the cause of my disease, wouldn't that mean that my emotions are especially toxic or problematic? Wouldn't that mean that if I could just control my emotions, I would be able to control my illness?"*

Perhaps worst of all, we think it means we are not actually sick and our symptoms are "imaginary." This idea may in part arise from the misunderstanding associated with psychosomatic illness—illness that is derived from the emotions or the mind. The term "psychosomatic" is often used when normal medical tests do not reveal the answer to an illness. It is usually regarded pejoratively, as something that is not entirely "real." The common treatment for issues that are emotional in origin is to take antidepressants.

The truth is, *every* disease is psychosomatic to one degree or another. You cannot separate your nervous system, your emotions, and your physical body from one another: they are connected! Everything we experience has an emotional as well as a physical basis, and the two deeply affect one another. Emotions affect the health of everyone.

According to Chinese medicine, the emotions, intellect, willpower, and spirit are housed throughout the body in all of the organs, not just in the brain or the heart. Healing, therefore, is holistic, and includes the emotions and the spirit since they are so deeply related and intertwined with the functioning of the body.

THE EMOTIONAL IMPACT

How many times have you had difficulty changing the way you feel? If we could flip a switch, most of us would just choose to be happy all of the time. The problem is, "control" can turn into suppression or blocking emotions, which leads to greater problems.

When a 5-year-old is angry, you know it. She screams, shouts, kicks, and makes a ruckus. She may even destroy something important to you or hurt you physically. For the 5-year-old, the temper tantrum is *very* intense while it is happening, but it is usually over in a matter of minutes.

As adults, we are expected to handle, process, and gracefully negotiate our emotions without being *affected* by them. When we express heightened emotionality, it is generally perceived as unprofessional, shameful, or weak —something to overcome or rein in. For most of us, rather than being completely honest and forthcoming about how we feel, we try to behave "appropriately." This means being "cool," not rocking the boat or making others feel uncomfortable. In the world and professionally, we separate ourselves from our emotions in order to feel we have more control in our lives.

If you suppress, ignore, or numb your emotions—or conversely, if you allow them to entirely dictate your life—it contributes to a blockage or disharmony in your energy flow. When your energy is blocked repeatedly, it begins to affect the body's ability to function optimally. Your life force energy, or *Qi*, is busy doing damage control, managing the stress factors or the blockages, rather than giving you vitality as it moves inside you. Remember: if you are ill, your body is simply and effectively signaling for you to pay attention to something while working to create more balance.

Fundamentals of the 5th Key
Emotions and Your Body

Ideally, we would all find ways to quickly process our emotions and maintain our health. The problem is, the emotions that make us sick are the same ones we hold most deeply inside ourselves. Often, those emotions are hidden and difficult to find, which is why they have not already been processed and released.

How do we begin to see emotions that are hidden? How do we

5th Key: Emotions and Your Body

> take responsibility without blaming ourselves or others? How do we address emotions that are so deep they are manifesting as symptoms in our bodies? And how do we feel safe in this process of discovery?
>
> The 5th Key, Emotions and Your Body, involves understanding how your emotions affect your physical health, and learning how to work with them. It is not psychotherapy, although psychotherapy can be a helpful tool in this process. The 5th Key is about understanding where and how your emotions originate so that you may better captain your responses. Ultimately, the fundamentals of the 5th Key will help your emotions move through your body, heart, and mind more quickly, and give you greater emotional and physical freedom, helping you to heal.

1st Fundamental: The Impact of Emotions on Your Health

According to Chinese medicine, there is always an emotional component to illness. Physical symptoms have an emotional component and emotional issues generate a physical response. We put so much time and attention on caring for our physical health, but our emotional well-being must be equally nurtured and attended to if we are to create true physical health.

2nd Fundamental: Emotions and the Organ Systems

If you have a medical problem that you are unable to easily resolve, explore the emotional aspect. In Chinese medicine, each of the major organ systems are ruled by a specific emotion. You can use this information to understand your body's issues. Through your body, you can discover the emotional root to your illness.

3rd Fundamental: Stress and Your Health
Stress is universally recognized as one of the greatest contributors to health problems. Even though stress is not always a bad thing, the stress that most of us experience from day to day can take a toll on our body and health. The best remedy for stress is finding a way to grow your love and joy.

4th Fundamental: Awareness: Cultivating the Observer
Learning to observe and identify your emotions has tremendous benefits to your physical health and overall well-being. Remember, you are not your emotions; they do not control or define you.

5th Fundamental: The Art of Taking Charge
There are specific physical actions you can take to create more emotional stability and strength. Being more emotionally grounded and clear also benefits your physical health and well-being on every level.

1st Fundamental
The Impact of Emotions on Your Health

Emotions are as significant to physical health as lifestyle and genetics.

I recognized at an early age that my emotions absolutely affected how I felt physically. This is part of the reason that Chinese medicine resonated so deeply with me. I was a "believer" in Chinese medicine before I even knew it existed!

My teenage years were extremely stressful. My stepfather had a personality disorder and had random bursts of violent anger, so we could never predict his behavior. My mother avoided any mention of his insanity and pretended

5th Key: Emotions and Your Body

that everything was OK, so my home life was nearly intolerable. Every night at dinner we would not know what was going to happen. Sometimes cold and uncommunicative, sometimes angry and violent, my stepfather's instability created an environment of constant stress for the whole family.

At 15, I started having pain in my left knee, which made it hard for me to walk. I had a paper route, so I was walking up and down hills every day. What began as a minor soreness in my knee became worse and worse until it was so painful that I needed surgery for a torn meniscus.

The week I spent in the hospital after my surgery turned out to be a huge blessing—I was able to escape my family for a few days! After I was discharged from the hospital, my knee did not heal properly in spite of intensive physical therapy and effort on my part. I continued to have pain for about a year. Throughout that year, whenever my knee pain was particularly bad, my mother and stepfather would leave me alone in my room. Even though the physical pain was terrible, my solitude, and not having to navigate my insufferable family dynamics, was a saving grace.

About a year after the surgery my doctor discovered that my meniscus, which had been "removed completely" in the surgery, and was not supposed to grow back, had actually grown back! This discovery showed me two things: 1) The body can heal, even when medicine says that it cannot; and 2) Science is not always accurate.

Since I was in pain, my doctors recommended that I have another operation, but I decided not to go through with it. The first operation had not solved the issue, so I did not see how having a second operation would be more effective. I didn't want to go through that kind of pain again for no change in outcome.

Throughout this experience, I realized that my knee pain was largely connected to the stress in my family life. It was then that I started to make the connection, and understand that my emotions must be playing a part in how my body felt. Of course, I didn't think about it directly at the time. After

I graduated from high school my mom and stepfather separated, and my stepfather moved away. Remarkably, once he was gone, my knee pain went away completely!

THE ORIGINS OF ILLNESS—INNER AND OUTER

According to Chinese medicine, your emotions play a *huge* role in your overall health—as big as any other factor in your life. Your body is made up of energy, and emotions provide a way for energy to move in the body. Every time you have an experience, the energy from that experience needs to go somewhere. This is a basic law of physics—energy is neither created nor destroyed, but it can change form. So, when you have an argument with someone and you're angry, that experience translates into energy moving inside of you. Depending upon the intensity of the experience, your ability to process it, and how often that emotion is triggered, the emotional energy from your experiences can be stored and held in your physical body.

In Chinese medicine, illness is the product of blocked, disrupted, excessive or unbalanced energy movement *(Qi)* along the meridians of the body. Illness can originate either **outside the body,** through a trauma or infection, or **inside the body,** through an emotional imbalance. When you become sick, your body is signaling that there is an imbalance—a blockage, a weakening, or an excess of energy. Too much of one emotion, or unexpressed or suppressed emotions, weakens the *Qi* and causes illness.

Let's say something happened to you when you were a kid. Maybe you were told that you weren't smart or good enough. Maybe you didn't feel safe in your home. Those experiences are a part of your upbringing, so those feelings become "normal." Rather than being in a constant state of emotional pain, you suppress your emotions. Your emotions begin to affect your body physically. You may not even realize that you have emotional stress until it begins to manifest in your body and even then, it can look like a physical problem, not connected to emotions at all.

5th Key: Emotions and Your Body

I've mentioned the ACE (Adverse Childhood Events) study before (Felitti, Anda, et. al 1998), which documents that the more ACE a person has, the more they are prone to physical illness, emotional imbalance, and early death. Since the original study was done in 1998, more than 50 additional studies have corroborated that information.

We constantly experience emotions, and they embed themselves in our bodies. Many factors, including physical strength, family history, genetics, and overall health play a role in how your body handles the energy and emotions you are storing. The good news is, by becoming aware that your emotions play a role in your health, you can begin to change how your emotions affect you.

The Way It Works

When your feelings are hurt, or when you are emotionally impacted by an experience, you may not even notice that it happened. You may be so used to brushing it aside, or handling things a certain way that you may not notice what happened to your body in response to that event. What I know from my own experiences and from many years of working with patients, is that if you do not resolve the emotional angst, it will come up again in some other way. This is not to say that every current or past conflict is living in your body somewhere, but there are deep wounds that can take time to repair.

As an adult, you may have had a physical experience such as a massage, or a run, or a big crying session when you spontaneously recalled certain buried feelings or memories from your past. In such instances, your body may have been holding onto those experiences, or the emotions from them, until just that moment when you were able to release them.

Have you ever caught a cold after a particularly emotional experience, such as after you've had a fight with a loved one? Sometimes, an illness can actually help you *purge* certain emotions you've been holding in for a long time.

Other times, an emotion can be the *cause* of a physical issue. Repressed anger can cause neck tension, and it can also rise up into the head, leading to hypertension or migraines. The liver regulates the emotion of anger, the smooth flow of energy in the whole body, and the ligaments and tendons. Anger held in the body can be like a pressure cooker. It is a hot energy, and needs someplace to go, so if held in too long, it can lead to many physical symptoms. This is also true of the other organs, such as the spleen, which rules your digestion and the emotion of worry. Excessive worry can lead to stomach problems. The lungs rule the emotion of grief, so when you're going through grief, you might get lung congestion, or a cough, or a flu.

During my fourth year of medical school, before I knew anything about Chinese medicine, I broke up with my longtime boyfriend. After we broke up, I was sick for a few days with a cold, but afterward I continued to cough for several months. My roommate at the time (who was also a med student) wanted me to be tested for TB because I coughed so much! Years later, I learned that lungs are associated with the emotion of grief, and I realized that coughing was the way that my body had helped me release the emotions about my relationship.

An injury can also affect the emotional and spiritual aspects that are associated with that organ. For example, if you sprain your ankle, and the location of the sprain is in the liver meridian, you may experience added frustration while it heals, since the liver is associated with anger. Everything is interconnected.

TRAUMA—PTSD

JOEY

Joey was 16 years old when he was assaulted by school bullies. He wasn't physically injured because the police arrived, but shortly after the event, he began to be very irritable with his parents. He easily lost control of his temper. At first,

5th Key: Emotions and Your Body

everyone thought he was just being a teenager, but when he became violent unexpectedly, they realized something was wrong. When his parents brought him to my office and explained what had happened, I treated him for PTSD using acupuncture. Within a few weeks, he began to feel more like his old self again.

When a person experiences something that deeply affects them on an emotional or spiritual level, it can create an energy imbalance that may or may not develop into PTSD. Allergies, asthma, digestive problems, sleep problems, depression, and anxiety are all symptoms that can come from PTSD.

An estimated 70 percent of Americans have experienced a traumatic event at least one time in their life. (Felitti, Anda, et. al 1998.) If you experience emotional trauma, your body will either heal itself or continue to have an energy blockage as a result of that event. You may develop certain behavior patterns, or you may become physically ill.

Any type of trauma can create an energy blockage, which can deeply affect us. If we are in a car accident, for example, the physical trauma is apparent, and we immediately work to address the physical symptoms. Emotional trauma can have a similar sudden intense impact, much like a car accident, but because we tend to ignore our emotions, we are often not aware of the emotional impact, and therefore do not immediately and urgently address it.

The brain is affected in many ways as a result of trauma, which influences our behavior and ability to function. If you have any of the following symptoms, you may be suffering from PTSD:
- Inability to regulate emotions
- Short-term memory loss
- Constant feel of fright
- Need for isolation
- Trouble sleeping
- Sudden increase in physical symptoms

If you feel you may be suffering from PTSD, you should seek professional help. Don't be afraid to say how you are feeling, and that you need help. After all, good health and well-being is our greatest asset, and we need our body and mind to last an entire lifetime. Acupuncture is a great complementary technique for resolving many issues connected to PTSD.

Actions and Exercises for the 1st Fundamental
The Impact of Emotions on Your Health

Releasing Emotions

The actions for the 1st Fundamental are all about learning to process and release your emotions quickly. This helps them move through your body and promotes balanced Qi and good health. Below are a few basic techniques that can help.

1. **Immediate Release**

    Crying, laughing, shouting, and singing are all ways to immediately move energy and re-establish balance in your body. Don't be afraid to express yourself. And, whenever possible, do it immediately upon experiencing the emotion.

2. **Creative Release**

    Look for creative ways to process your experiences. Your anger may turn into an amazing workout session. Your sadness may turn into a beautiful poem or a song. Your joy may become an offering of a meal or gifts to loved ones. Your fear may motivate you to find the tools that you need to navigate stressful situations. Tap into the energy that your emotions give to you and *do something* with it.

3. **Talking It Out**

   Expressing how you feel, without blame or becoming a victim, is a very healing way to become more self-aware of your feelings. Talk to your friends and family. Find people who have had similar experiences and who can relate to what you are going through.

4. **Distraction**

   Have you ever used distraction to manage an energetic child or a romping pet? You can try the same thing on yourself! Sometimes, a little distraction is exactly what you need to shift from feeling bad to feeling better.

5. **Focus on It**

   When you experience an emotion, don't run away from it. Instead, allow it to happen. Focus all your attention on experiencing that feeling. You can even try to hold onto it! You may find when you do that, it will dissipate more readily.

6. **A Good Read**

   Peter Levine's book, *Healing Trauma: A Pioneering Program for Restoring the Wisdom of your Body*, talks about how animals are able to literally "shake off" the experience of a trauma in order to release the energy that their body has generated when threatened. He claims that people lose their ground during trauma, and that becoming grounded is the way to deal with our emotions.

2nd Fundamental
Emotions and the Organ Systems

SHARON

Sharon came to me with chronic sinus infections. She was 32 years old when the infections began. She had been having three to four episodes per year for the past three years, and it never completely cleared up between. She had been on multiple courses of antibiotics, was using steroid nasal sprays, and doing nasal washes, but nothing was making her sinus infections better.

During her initial visit, Sharon told me that when she was 29 years old, her brother had died of leukemia. He was one of her best friends. In Chinese medicine, the lungs rule the emotion of grief, and their spiritual function is to keep you in your physical body. They also protect you from things that come in from outside and are connected to your immune system. The lungs rule the entire respiratory system including your nose, throat, and lungs. When grief is deep, it is not unusual to have some sort of respiratory illness. I've seen this literally hundreds of times in my practice.

Sharon had not been able to overcome the grief of losing her brother but hadn't really been aware how much it affected her. As we did a series of acupuncture treatments and supplements to restore her immune system, Sharon healed.

I love acupuncture because it allows me to help a person emotionally, even when they don't fully know or understand where the emotions are coming from. Part of Sharon's healing involved understanding that her grief was connected to her physical illness. This awareness allowed her to create a shift in herself, which supported the healing she received from acupuncture and nutritional supplements. It's been ten years since we were able to restore her immune system to balance, and Sharon has not had another sinus infection since.

5th Key: Emotions and Your Body

As you've already learned, specific emotions are connected to each of the organ systems, and these connections make a lot of sense. Grief is connected to the lungs, so when we cry, it is our lungs and chest that feel the experience. When we worry about something, we usually have knots in our stomach and difficulty eating. Worry is connected to the stomach and the spleen. When we experience joy, we feel it in our heart. The heart is ruled by joy.

Perhaps the most important thing to do with the 5th Key is to simply understand that there is an emotional connection to how you feel physically. By becoming aware of your emotional tendencies, you may then understand which organ is more likely to go out of balance. What is the dominant emotion you experience on a regular basis? Is it sadness? Anger? Anxiety? Fear? Excitement? For much of my life I had a tendency to be angry, so I had a lot of liver symptoms, including migraines, menstrual cramps, tight neck and shoulders and irritable bowel syndrome (the liver can affect the digestive system because it is in charge of the smooth flow of energy in all of the organs).

The next section explains how each organ works in Chinese medicine, and which emotion is connected to each organ. By understanding this, you will be able to understand some of the ways in which emotions can affect your health, or vice versa. This is one secret to understanding your own body. With this information, you can learn how to approach your healing and perhaps begin to understand the emotional roots behind your health concerns.

HEART AND SMALL INTESTINES: JOY

The heart and small intestines rule the emotion of Joy. The heart pumps blood and gives sustenance to all the organs, so it is seen to be in command. When the heart is strong, it controls the emotions. When it is weak, the emotions rebel.

The small intestine's job is to separate the clear from the turbid, a function which relates to digestion but also has to do with the ability to discern clear from turbid thoughts, actions, and emotions. The small intestine meridian travels across the shoulder blade—often a person might have a shoulder pain when her small intestine meridian is irritated, which might also manifest in an inability to think clearly about some things. By understanding this, you might be able to figure out a way to balance the small intestine and support clear thinking, which would then help heal the shoulder pain.

An overabundance of joy sounds like a good thing, but excitability and mania scatters Qi. Extreme joy is mania. Because the tongue is the root of the heart, talking incessantly, laughing inappropriately, or, on the opposite end, an inability to speak or other speech problems, can all be signs of an imbalance in the heart. Dysfunctions of the heart can cause mental restlessness, poor memory, depression, anxiety, and insomnia.

Excessive craving and addiction can also be an aspect of joy—or more precisely, a *lack of joy*. When we obsessively seek happiness, it creates an imbalance that may show up as an addiction, and addictions do not provide the fulfillment we crave.

Pure joy—delight in life—is *balanced* heart energy.

ACTIONS FOR THE HEART
- Smiling stimulates the heart. Watch a funny movie so that you can laugh. Or, just laugh for no reason. Make other people laugh. Try to laugh every day.
- Put your hands upon your heart and just feel it beating. Bring your awareness to the power of your heart.
- There are a few yoga poses that are particularly great for opening the heart: Cobra and Upward dog are two poses that expand your chest and heart center. Another good one is to clasp your hands behind your back and bend forward from the hips and hang like a rag doll with your arms moving toward the floor.

5th Key: Emotions and Your Body

LUNGS AND LARGE INTESTINES: GRIEF

The lungs and large intestines rule the emotion of grief. They are connected to the immune system, the skin, and the nose. They are the outermost layer of your energy. They protect the interior, so when you become sick, it often means that your lungs are weakened.

When we cry, our lungs are affected. Grief depresses and weakens the lungs, and prolonged grief or unexpressed grief weakens the lung Qi—which can lead to such things as chronic asthma, bronchitis, irritable bowel syndrome, or chronic diarrhea. If you're hanging on to emotions, it may cause constipation or even symptoms of irritable bowel syndrome.

If you are experiencing issues with your lungs or immune system, or you have felt intense or prolonged sadness or grief, spend some time paying attention to your breath. Breathing deeply is one very simple thing that you can do to relax your nervous system and strengthen your Lung Qi.

ACTIONS FOR THE LUNGS
Deep Breathing Exercises

- Try alternate nostril breathing, which is a powerful Yogic breathing practice. Simply take your right hand and close your right nostril with your thumb. Exhale slowly until all of your breath is released. Then, inhale slowly, keeping your thumb on your right nostril. Once you are at the top of your breath, release your thumb from your right nostril and close your left nostril with your ring finger. Exhale slowly, then inhale, keeping your left nostril closed and filling your lungs and belly completely. At the top of that breath, switch back to your thumb and right nostril.

    Try doing this for just two minutes a day. See how your emotions, your nervous system, and your body feel when you are finished. After one week, notice if there is a difference in how you feel emotionally.

- If you have recently lost a loved one—either through death or separation—try spending some time each day, for a few minutes, in reflection. I think of the Jewish ritual of sitting Shiva for a week after someone has died, which allows a family to process the grief together. If you have suffered a loss, I recommend spending some dedicated time to allow the grief to run through you. It might help prevent physical issues in the future.
- Yoga Pose for the Large Intestines: There's a yoga pose called the Garland or *Malasana* pose, where you sit on your heels with feet slightly wider than hips width apart, and squat down, resting your elbows on the inside of your knees, with your hands at your heart. Do this for one minute a day; it will help connect you to the earth, open your pelvis, lower back, and sphincter muscle, increase hip flexibility, and becomes a great resting pose.

SPLEEN AND STOMACH: WORRY, PENSIVENESS

The spleen and stomach rule the emotion of worry. Their job is to take in food, transform that food into energy, and transport that energy to the lungs, which will then circulate the "gu" Qi (energy of food) to the rest of the body. The spleen is connected to the muscles in your body and to your lips. This is the organ system most affected by what you eat, and how you eat. Therefore, it responds well to changes in diet.

If you find yourself compulsively overthinking things, or anxious all of the time, you may want to consider finding ways to support your stomach and spleen. I have had countless patients who experience anxiety, and part of it comes from their diet. Too much caffeine, sugar, and processed foods can contribute to physical and emotional imbalances. Something as simple as cutting back on your caffeine intake may greatly impact your overall anxiety.

5th Key: Emotions and Your Body

ACTIONS FOR THE SPLEEN
- To support the stomach and spleen, eat cooked, warm foods. It is easier to digest cooked food. Smaller, more frequent meals can also be less taxing on the stomach and spleen. Interestingly, if you have a weak spleen, raw food will not be good for you (even though it seems so healthy!) because your body won't be able to properly transform it into energy.
- If you tend to worry a lot, certain foods are good for your spleen: sweet potatoes, butternut squash, steamed carrots, cinnamon, dates, and lentils. Eating them can help you feel calmer.
- High quality protein in your diet will also help you feel more grounded and better because it helps balance your blood sugar and keeps it more stable.
- Yoga poses to counteract worry and anxiousness:
  - Tree pose (connecting to the earth)
  - Boat pose (arms and legs in a V, working abs)

LIVER AND GALL BLADDER: ANGER

The liver and the gallbladder rule the emotion of anger. The liver is connected to the eyes and regulates the menstrual cycles and the ligaments and tendons. One of the main jobs of the liver is to insure the smooth flow of Qi throughout the body. When our energy is obstructed (or frustrated) the liver is affected. The liver, therefore, is greatly affected by stress.

Anger makes the Qi rise, so anger is experienced physically in our head and neck, with headaches, or a red, blotchy face,

ACTIONS FOR THE LIVER
- Sweating and exercise aid in liver detoxification, so the best thing you can do when you are angry, or dealing with a liver imbalance, is to be diligent with an exercise routine. To immediately release

feelings of anger you can do 50 jumping jacks or 20 push-ups. This is a quick and drama-free way to move anger out of your body.
- Yoga pose for Anger:
    - Warrior I (lateral and medial parts of the body)
- Leafy greens are good for the liver and when you want to support it, you can eat a lot of them. If you are having anger or liver symptoms, you can avoid drinking alcohol, and eating fatty, processed foods.

KIDNEY AND URINARY BLADDER: FEAR

According to Chinese medicine, the kidneys rule the emotion of fear. Kidneys hold our Qi, our essence, and are the root of our sexuality and energy. The kidneys are connected to the ears and the bones.

Our kidneys give us our overall sense of energy. Sexuality, libido, and creativity are all associated with the kidneys. It is thought that fear depletes our Qi. Chronic low-grade fear translates to stress and deeply affects the kidneys.

ACTIONS FOR THE KIDNEYS

- If you feel a lot of fear, especially fear for no apparent reason, try doing something a little scary. Maybe go to a class by yourself: stretch beyond your comfort zone. Take small steps, but try to do something that's a little frightening at least once a week.
- This is a helpful meditation to help you relax your fear: Inhale, and imagine yourself surrounded by love and light. Exhale, and imagine you are exhaling your fear.
- Yoga pose for Fear:
    - Bow pose (laying on your stomach—massaging kidneys)

3rd Fundamental
Stress and Your Health

POSITIVE STRESS

The CDC estimates that stress accounts for 75% of all doctors visits (Mohd, Malay J. Med.Sci, 2008) Chronic stress, which often manifests as anger or anxiety, alters the heart's electrical stability, increases systemic inflammation, and raises hypertension and blood cholesterol in adults. (Torpy, Lymn, Glass, JAMA, 2007). Emotional distress and its side effects—including disturbed sleep, digestive problems, and muscular pain—can weaken the body and make it more susceptible to disease. When we are stressed, something that would naturally heal may linger as malaise, and it can even cause conditions to relapse, like knee pain, or a recurrent sore throat.

It's not surprising that emotional stress is now considered a major contributing factor in the six leading causes of death in the US. That list includes cancer, heart disease, accidental injuries, respiratory disorders, cirrhosis of the liver, and suicide. (Mohd, Razalli, Saleh, 2008)

Stress, however, is not universally bad. It is a necessary part of human survival and it is one of the things that helps us grow. Studies have shown that short-term stress can even boost our immune system. (Ratue, 2012) The "fight or flight" response (which is the stress response in our bodies) compels us to adapt and respond appropriately to danger. We often feel most motivated and work best under pressure. This is the kind of stress that professional athletes, performers, and college students in the throes of exams might use to excel.

Stress is positive when it propels us to change—when it causes us to push ourselves to meet a challenge. Stress becomes problematic when it is chronic—when we are in a constant state of overdrive. This damaging stress can harm our health and deplete our immune system. Long-term and persistent stress causes too much wear and tear on the system and makes us more susceptible to illness.

Stress is positive when it propels us to change—when it causes us to push ourselves to meet a challenge. Stress becomes problematic when it is chronic—when we are in a constant state of overdrive—or when we feel that we don't have the capacity to handle our problems. This damaging stress can harm our health and deplete our immune system. Long term and persistent stress causes too much wear and tear on the system, and makes us more susceptible to illness.

A study by professor of psychiatry, M.R. Salleh, in 2008, revealed that our attitude toward our experiences, including our feeling that things will improve and that we can handle our problems, is the greatest determinant of our stress level and our overall health. He showed that when someone experiences an extreme trauma, and sees it as meaningful, they are healthier and less stressed than the person who does not experience trauma, but who has an overall sense of futility or despair about their life. Therefore, people who feel that their lives have meaning, no matter their circumstances, are more physically healthy than those who feel their lives are meaningless. If you see stress as a motivator and an opportunity to grow, learn and improve, stress can actually increase your longevity.

It is always good to try to reduce the stress in your life, but in relationship to your body, if you feel that you are at the mercy of an illness, your body will experience more negative stress. If you believe that *you can heal,* and that you are growing through your experiences, your overall stress will be reduced and your immune system can be strengthened.

THE POSITIVE SIDE OF NEGATIVE THINKING

Interestingly, believing that you can heal does not mean that you need to "think positively" about your condition in order to heal. In his book, *When the Body Says No,* Dr. Gabor Maté explores the emotional roots of severe illness. He found that *appropriate* negative thinking was actually helpful in healing.

This means that, while we are always moving toward our goal of healing, we also give ourselves permission to honestly acknowledge the difficulties we face. Sometimes we need to explore the darkest places in order to bring in the light. People often suppress traumas or pain and don't recognize that their desire to only be "positive" may be preventing them from seeing the truth about their past. If we don't recognize what is challenging about our situation, we may be denying or suppressing certain very real emotions which inevitably affects our bodies.

For example, my patient Denise has always been super positive about her process, to the extent that she has become scattered, almost manic, in her communication. She avoided looking at what was negative about her experiences by being constantly positive. The truth is, when you are sick, there are certain *facts* that just are not great. I spoke to Denise about this, because she was dealing with some severe physical issues, and I felt that her constant "Miss Positive" attitude was creating an imbalance, which could potentially impede her healing.

Being honest with yourself about the severity of your condition, and acknowledging the parts of you that are struggling with negativity and hopelessness, allows those emotions and thoughts to be released and not held in your body. The trick is to not become mired in your pain, to keep moving forward, and to find ways to redirect your thoughts *toward what is possible.*

Healing When It Seems Impossible

Actions and Exercises for the 3rd Fundamental Understanding Stress

1. **Replace!**
   You can't just eliminate your negative thoughts. To do so would most likely be denying very real emotions and thoughts. The point, instead, is to work to replace them. For example, if you find yourself thinking "I'm never going to heal. This is never going to end." Say to yourself "My body is my friend. My body is capable of healing."

2. **Look at the Negative Thoughts—Really Look at Them**
   Make a list of the reasons why you think you'll never heal, why you feel afraid, what makes you feel hopeless or angry. Give yourself time for this exercise—spend a week or two really exploring the part of you that doesn't think you can make it, that feels that it's unfair, that feels betrayed, that wants to give up. Then, figure out what you really want, and move toward that goal.

4th Fundamental
Awareness—Cultivating the Observer

BRIAN

My patient Brian was 37 years old and a firefighter. He came to see me because he was experiencing terrible knee pain. He had been dealing with the pain for a year, and he didn't want to have surgery.

Brian received acupuncture from me, but it wasn't solving the problem.

5th Key: Emotions and Your Body

From my experience, when a physical problem is not improving with treatment then it's time to ask: "Is there something else going on?" I asked Brian if there was anything in his life that was causing him stress, or that didn't feel good. Brian was married with two kids and a busy life, but he kept telling me that everything was great, that he didn't have any problems.

Then one day, he happened to mention that he had just had lunch with his father. I asked him, "How was it?" He said, "Oh, well, my dad's an alcoholic."

Alarm bells rang in my head. I told him that having an alcoholic family member can affect a person's life, including his emotional well-being. I explained that the pain in his knee was along his gall bladder meridian, which has to do with anger and frustration. It was also on his right side, which is the masculine side (the right side of the body is commonly considered the masculine or expressing side, whereas the left side of the body is considered the feminine or receiving side). To take it a bit further, the knees are a part of the first chakra, the root chakra, which has to do with our connection with our tribe and our sense of safety and security in the world.

When I shared this information with Brian, it completely changed his life. The fact that his upbringing and his emotions could have affected him physically made him curious. He began to read books, and eventually he went into therapy. It was then, after he began to address his emotions, that his knee started to respond to acupuncture.

Awareness

In Zen Buddhism there is a meditation practice called *Zazen*. It is concerned with observing the mind, and not being attached to the thoughts and concepts that pass through it. When people are able to achieve this state of mind, they experience great relaxation and a sense of letting go.

This practice of creating the "observer" is prevalent in many spiritual practices, and for good reason. It is human to be reactive, but what once served to protect us—our ability to react quickly when threatened—is no longer necessary for our survival. Yet, our reactiveness remains, innate in our psyche. Changing those thinking patterns is hard work. It requires diligence and a consistent approach.

You can begin creating awareness of your emotions simply by *noticing* them. By learning to observe your emotions, you develop a greater capacity to have a more objective perspective. When you have a strong emotional reaction, try saying: "Wow! I am very (angry, sad, hurt) right now." From this viewpoint you may notice that you can discern with more clarity what you are feeling, and why you are feeling that way.

Also, pay attention to where you are feeling certain emotions in your body. Literally, *where do you feel the emotion?* We talk about emotions as feelings, because they show up in our body—but so often people don't understand their "feelings". I had a patient who experienced anger simply as a tingling in her scalp. She often wasn't aware of the emotion otherwise, but past experiences helped her understand that when her head tingled she was experiencing anger. Anger makes the *Qi* rise, so we often feel it in our heads and faces.

Without knowing it, she was reading her body in order to understand her emotions. If you can begin to pay attention to your body—how and where you are feeling things in your body—you might be able to better understand yourself emotionally, and be able to handle your emotions before they reach a more critical point.

Awareness allows emotions to move through your body with greater ease, and more quickly. When you become more objectively aware of what you are feeling, you'll have more emotional flexibility, and therefore, more choices and resources available. Eventually, awareness can help you choose *how* to respond. You'll still experience your emotions, but you'll feel more in charge, and not as reactive.

5th Key: Emotions and Your Body

Actions and Exercises for the 4th Fundamental Awareness—Cultivating the Observer

1. **Practice Being the Observer**
   - As a meditation, set a timer and spend 3-5 minutes a day observing your thoughts.
   - Do not judge them, do not attempt to stop or change them, just *watch* what you are thinking and feeling. Allow your thoughts to move through your mind, like a movie.
   - This practice helps you realize that your thoughts and feelings do not define you, they are just a part of you. You can watch them, and thereby learn to take charge of them.

2. **Be Your Own Hunter**
   - Recall the last time you had a strong emotional response to something or someone: How did your body feel? Where did you feel the emotion in your body?
   - What did you do to deal with those sensations in your body?
   - What did you do afterward? Did you verbally express yourself? Did you exercise? Did you eat? Did you turn on the TV? Did you have sex?
   - Did it bother you the next day or did it remedy itself in the moment?
   - What did your self-talk sound like?
   - Did the emotion start out as one thing, and then turn into another emotion? Often, sadness turns into anger upon contemplation (or vice versa).

- Keep a journal about these experiences and insights. Notice any patterns and make note of successes!

3. **Exploration:** What foods do you crave and when do you crave them? What are your thoughts around certain emotions? What memories and smells do you connect to specific emotions? Are your thoughts a part of your conditioning, or are they coming from someplace deeper inside of you? How do you *feel*—right now? You can learn so much about yourself just by taking the time to *observe*.

5th Fundamental
Taking Charge of Your Emotions

CARRIE

My patient Carrie has multiple sclerosis, breast cancer, and sleep problems. When she first came to see me, she was taking 40 different supplements, several medications, and had received chemotherapy, radiation, and surgery for her cancer. Carrie had seven different doctors and had been working on the physical and lifestyle aspects of her illnesses for years, but she still felt really sick most of the time.

In spite of her diligent work to heal herself on a physical level, Carrie had not explored the impact of her emotions on her body before she came to see me. She told me that the idea of taking pain pills for the rest of her life was horrifying to her. She was ready to do anything. She was ready to change on a fundamental level.

After we discussed the possibility that there could be an emotional element that was affecting her health, Carrie began to explore how she felt. She realized that she was angry about everything. Her marriage was not what she wanted, her career was unsatisfying, and she was completely overwhelmed with the duties of taking care of her very demanding and ailing parents.

The best way to release anger is through physical exertion. Carrie had a hard time exercising because she was so exhausted due to her physical conditions. I suggested that she begin by walking a little each day, and as she walked, to focus upon all the things that made her angry. She learned to use her breath and the physical movement of exercise to begin consciously releasing her emotions so they would not be stuck in her body.

Slowly, as she began moving her body and expressing her emotions, she began to feel better. She began to have more energy so she could exercise more. She decided to retire from her job. After a while, she saw that her husband did love her, he just expressed how he loved her differently than what she had expected over the years. They began to communicate more as she healed, and their relationship began to improve. As her healing progressed, she realized that she felt less exhausted.

Over the course of several months Carrie had more and more energy, less pain, and was able to go off her medications. She and her husband created a deeper connection and even ended up going on an exotic second honeymoon. By being open to addressing her emotional well-being as a part of her health regime, every element of her life improved.

You Are Not Your Emotions

There is great freedom in recognizing that your emotions are a just a part of your experience. YOU are not your emotions. Your emotions do not define or control you. They are a response, a signal for you to pay attention.

By becoming less identified with your emotional response, you can respond in a more loving way. You can be generous, even in the face of feeling deprived. You can be kind, even when you feel that someone has hurt you. These responses, the response of kindness and love, generate kindness and love. So, rather than perpetuating a cycle of anger, or sadness, or fear, you are breaking that cycle and beginning something new, transformative, and healing.

You may notice that as your body becomes stronger through attention to lifestyle and physical support, your emotions seem heightened. Like Carrie, perhaps now that you've worked to open yourself up physically, your emotions are able to rise to the surface and move through you more readily. This is a good thing.

PHYSICALLY RELEASING EMOTIONS

Your body is this great processor for your emotions, but you can also help to physically facilitate emotional release. Exercise helps process your emotions and clears your head. It is universally beneficial because physical movement changes the energy and emotions that you are storing in your body. Often, simply by moving your body, you can receive more clarity about how you feel. Exercising regularly is an essential part of the 3rd Key—Lifestyle—but it is equally important for the 5th Key, as it helps to create emotional stability, strength, and clarity.

Specific healing modalities can help release emotions. Acupuncture, massage, other forms of bodywork, and even a hot shower can do a world of good to release stuck emotions. In addition, the following physical and mental exercises can help facilitate emotional release.

Actions for the 5th Fundamental
Taking Charge of Your Emotions

1. **Exercise:** Think of exercise as medicine. Hiking along a nature trail, bicycling down a winding road, visiting the gym, or dancing to a favorite song will raise your heart rate, generate endorphins, and remind you that

5th Key: Emotions and Your Body

there is a larger world outside your inner turmoil.

When you are feeling emotional, try moving your body physically to discharge the energy. You can try jumping jacks, push-ups, or climbing a big hill—anything that gets your body moving and your blood pumping. If you are in an environment (like work) where you can't drop and do 20 push-ups, try clenching the muscles in your hands, butt, and/or perineum, and then relaxing those muscles. Repeat as necessary.

2. **Sleep:** Like exercise, sleep clears the mind, opens up channels of understanding, and facilitates mental clarity. When you are rested, you may be better able to understand how you feel, and from where your emotions originate.

3. **Breathing:** Deep breathing works wonders for relaxing your body and releasing pent-up emotions. Coughing is also a great way to release emotions since so much emotion has to do with grief. So if you find yourself laughing to the point of coughing, you are doing more than just working out your lungs—you are actually releasing old emotions!

4. **Diet:** What you eat largely influences how you process emotions. Many people are negatively affected on an emotional level by sugar and carbohydrates. Therefore, if you eat in a healthy way, with lots of vegetables, protein, and healthy fats, you may find that you are more grounded and stable on an emotional level. You may be less likely to be triggered and irritable. Eating healthy foods doesn't specifically help you *process* emotions, but it lays the foundation for your whole body to be able to function with greater ease.

5. **Supplements:** You can support your body with supplements. Hormones and neurotransmitters (the signaling chemicals from your brain) have a

huge effect on our emotional state, and both can be greatly influenced by taking daily supplements. There is now a simple urine test that allows us to measure chemicals produced by the brain, and with these results, we can take natural supplements to help the brain achieve better balance.

6. **Mentally track down the root of your emotional distress:** If you are unsure why you are feeling a certain way, or maybe you don't understand *what you are feeling*, try looking at your emotions from a mental standpoint. *Why* are you upset? What triggered it? When did it begin? You may find that the roots of many of your painful emotions are connected to the same basic trigger. For example, you may have an old pain connected to rejection, or the pain of being left alone.

    Once you discover the logical root of your emotions, you may find relief and release of that emotion, as well as more compassion for yourself.

    You don't need to uncover specific emotional traumas from the past in order to understand the origin of your hurt feelings. Childhood memories are just memories—it is the way you feel that needs attention. An experience or some sort of conditioning from your past can cause you to respond to situations in a certain way. By recognizing these deep and long-held reactive and default thoughts or emotions inside of you, you can bring more consciousness to your present experiences, and have more choice about responding, rather than reacting.

Chapter 6

6th Key: Never Give Up! Patience and Persistence

"A hero is no braver than an ordinary man, but he is brave five minutes longer."
—Ralph Waldo Emerson

Julia

Julia was 60 when I first met her and she had been experiencing terrible vertigo for about a year. Prior to meeting me, she had found a dentist who worked to align her jaw and had been seeing a chiropractor, and both techniques had helped her significantly, but she still felt exhausted and overwhelmed by her symptoms. One of her worst symptoms was fatigue—she felt weak, tired, and anxious all of the time.

I gave Julia acupuncture and worked on balancing her hormones and brain chemistry, which helped her overall energy. Through the course of our work together, Julia began to heal but she still had significant times of fatigue, which really upset her.

Over the course of working with Julia, she told me that when she was an infant, her mother had TB and was sent to a sanitarium to convalesce. This experience deeply affected Julia.

Of course, she was too young to understand why her mother disappeared for 18 months, so she had felt abandoned. Even though her mother returned, Julia felt insecure, unsafe, and never truly loved throughout her life. She was never able to feel close to her mother and never felt that her mother loved her.

Julia was a go-getter. As a young mother, she was the mom who did everything. She was always busy taking care of everyone else, but her care-taking tendency stemmed from her own fear of instability.

We talked about how fear affects the adrenals. When we live in fear, we are constantly on the alert—in fight-or-flight mode. This hyper-vigilance can deplete the hormones that are made by the adrenals and can cause fatigue. Julia had become too tired to "run."

Julia and I worked together on her healing for four years, and in that time her symptoms became more manageable, but she still experienced occasional dizziness and fatigue. What was amazing about Julia is that despite feeling discouraged, and sometimes even hopeless, she never gave up. She always returned to her search, ready to try anything.

One day, Julia reached the peak of her frustration and fear about her vertigo. She became so upset that she ran to her husband and asked him to hold her. He did, and while he held her, she remembered a photo of her parents holding her, and looking at her with so much love. When her mother became ill she had lost her connection with her parents, and had always thought that they did not love her. In that moment, in her husband's arms, Julia realized that they had loved her—a lot.

When she came in to see me for her next session, Julia told me about this experience. I did my PTSD acupuncture treatments on her, and during one of those treatments she said that she realized she had never allowed her mother into her heart. Finally, though her parents had already passed, she was able to feel their love.

Through this healing she built her spiritual connection with her relatives and began to feel supported in her body in ways she never had before. Since then, she has not had the extreme fatigue or vertigo symptoms.

Julia recognizes that her life has transformed because of her illness. She knows that if she did not have extreme symptoms she would not have sought help. She would not have met all the people who helped her heal—not just in her body, but also in her heart. Each healing method gave her new tools to handle her symptoms. She feels her life is "bigger" now, and she has gained a healing that she can now share with others.

BECOMING THE HERO

> *"The most beautiful people we have known are those who have known defeat, known suffering, known struggle, known loss, and have found their way out of those depths."*
> —ELISABETH KUBLER-ROSS

In every Hero's journey, the Hero at some point encounters a trial so great that for a moment it seems all is lost and the goal is unattainable. That moment—when he finds a way to rise from his deepest doubts and fears and *act* with confidence and courage—is the moment when he becomes the Hero. In the stories, that is when we cheer the loudest, because we know those places of doubt inside of ourselves. We want the hero to make it, not just for the story, but for us. She helps us believe that the impossible is actually possible. The Hero symbolizes our hope for ourselves and our lives.

The healing path is a Hero's Journey, and the apex of that journey is the 6th Key. The 6th Key is about figuring out what stops us when things become difficult, and finding a way to break through those blocks and barriers. The 6th Key is finding a way to persevere even when the goal seems unattainable.

Like Odysseus, your journey may take longer than you expect. Like Perseus, you may encounter paralyzing foes. Like Luke Skywalker—and so many Heroes—you may not believe you are strong enough. And like Neo in *The Matrix*, you will find that the most powerful tools reside inside of you, and can be found through your heart.

Healing When It Seems Impossible

Crisis or Opportunity?

"When I dare to be powerful, to use my strength in the service of my vision, then it becomes less and less important whether I am afraid."
—Audre Lorde

The Chinese character for the word *crisis* is made up of two parts: one part represents *danger* and the other *opportunity*. When we approach a health crisis, or any crisis in life, it can be frightening and stressful, but it can also be an *opportunity* to transform.

Anytime you face a health crisis, it's like you're walking on a precipice. On one side you have everything to lose; on the other is your health, renewal, and a life that you love. The danger, which is what we generally focus on when we become sick, is that you could lose everything—even your life or your ability to function.

I know that the things that have challenged me the most in life are the very things that have taught me the most. Many of the difficulties I faced were physical problems. Those experiences made me look for solutions and helped me become a better doctor. I learned to be more present and compassionate with my patients, and *to never give up on the possibility for healing.*

One of the characteristics of the Hero is that she is willing to take on challenges. She *chooses* to leave her normal, ordinary world, and enter into an uncharted and magical land where the rules and limits are unknown. On our healing journeys, we all have the opportunity to cross into this field of adventure. From this new place, a crisis becomes an opportunity.

Our greatest challenges in life transform us. We may encounter these struggles and challenging places again and again. Each time the challenge can seem impossible, but we build our strength as we go. Our tenacity and resilience, and our ability to walk through these trials, again and again, make us the Hero of our own stories.

6th Key: Never Give Up! Patience and Persistence

> ## Fundamentals of the 6th Key
> ### *Patience and Persistence*
>
> The 6th Key is about overcoming challenges, preparing for those moments when you are knocked down, and summoning the will and the desire to persist, no matter what. No one can do this for you. Your allies, friends, family, healers and doctors can support you, but the desire to continue moving forward, and the fire to heal resides inside of you.

1st Fundamental: The Yin and Yang of Patience and Persistence
The pliable strength of patience and the force of persistence work together in harmony, like Yin and Yang. Both are needed to advance your health and healing, and they are vital to one another.

2nd Fundamental: Never Give Up!
A key factor to succeed in anything, including your healing, is a never-give-up attitude. We can cultivate this attitude by believing that our challenges actually help us grow, and that we absolutely have the ability and resources to achieve our goal.

3rd Fundamental: Divine Timing
Your body has its own perfect timing, and usually, healing takes time. Trust your body, and your process; avoid the yo-yo game of the "quick-fix."

4th Fundamental: Believe in Miracles
Some people think that a miracle is when you are cured of a deadly dis-

ease in an instant. But miracles are everywhere. Being able to recognize them boosts our mindset and our sense of hope. Miracles, big and small, are the gifts that we are all given on our healing journey.

5th Fundamental: Hope
Humans are designed to be hopeful—it is in our nature. At the same time, maintaining hope requires effort. When we are not eagerly striving toward our hope, it is just a fantasy, not grounded in reality.

1st Fundamental
The Yin and Yang of Patience & Persistence

"Do you have the patience to wait
Until your mud settles and the water is clear?
Can you remain unmoving
Until the right action arises by itself?"
—Lao Tzu (Tao Te Ching)

HEALING FROM EVERY ANGLE
As you now know, when I was 15 I had surgery on my left knee to repair a torn meniscus. As an adult, my right knee began troubling me after I overdid it with kickboxing and dancing. I had an MRI and discovered another torn meniscus! My doctor recommended surgery, but I decided to forego that option. It had not helped my other knee when I was young, and the pain of recovery was extreme. Instead, I wanted to use the information that I had received to heal myself.

I approached the issue with my knee from every possible angle. I received massage, acupuncture, and prolotherapy (which is an injection of a glucose solution into the area around the knee to initiate a healing response). I also did exercises to specifically help my knee. Emotionally, at the time, I felt that my husband did not respect my space. I found that when I expressed my needs and set clear boundaries, my knee pain would improve. Eventually when I was clear on my boundaries, it stopped being painful altogether.

My knee hurt for a long time—about 18 months. Of course I was stubborn and continued to exercise and COULD NOT resist dancing when great music was around. I listened, and waited, and persisted, and pushed. There were times when I thought that I would never see the end of the pain. There were times when I considered surgery. I also considered the possibility of living with the pain for the rest of my life.

Eventually, by examining my inner world, receiving support for my knee, being patient with the process and not giving up, my pain finally subsided. I couldn't say that there was any one thing that solved the issue. Everything contributed, and it was the process of working on my healing, patiently and persistently, that allowed my knee pain to be resolved.

COMMAND YOUR HEALTH

Patience and persistence balance one another—like Yin and Yang. Harmoniously, they support each other, and move us forward on our paths.

Persistence is fundamentally Yang. It embodies activities and functions, completes tasks, and is creative and logical, all of which are Yang qualities. Patience is fundamentally Yin, since it stores and transforms our energy. The Yin qualities of patience are intuitive, feminine, and nourishing.

Imagine the 6th Key is a boat on your healing journey. Persistence is the force and wind behind your actions. Patience is the anchor and the rudder. Patience sometimes directs the force, moving you from one location to the next, while other times, it holds steady, anchoring the action. You are the captain. You sit at the helm, taking command of your health.

Persistence—Yang

> *"Our greatest weakness lies in giving up. The most certain way to succeed is always to try just one more time."*
> —Thomas Edison

In health, persistence means looking for answers, trying different solutions, and being relentless in your search. It means the steadfast pursuit of your goal. Lack of persistence creates lethargy, victimhood, and oftentimes a feeling of failure.

We feel motivated to persist either when something is intolerable, or when we feel a commitment to a greater goal (for the sake of our children, family or community, for example). The will to persist relies in our belief that something good is going to come out of our efforts. Therefore, persistence is uniquely tied to hope.

Persistence needs patience, in the same way that Yang needs Yin. Otherwise, you may rush ahead and not allow something the time it needs to work.

Patience—Yin

Lenny

My patient Lenny had fibromyalgia. At 59, he was in so much pain he could not do the lifting required at his job as a grocery store stocker. When he used his arms, he was always achy. We used a combination of herbs, acupuncture, and diet to balance his body. After two months of working with me, he felt slightly better, but he was still in pain.

Lenny expressed his frustration to me and told me that he wanted to stop what we were doing because the results were still so slight. I encouraged him not to give up, and to allow the medicine the time that it needed to establish a new equilibrium in his body. After three more months, he was a different person. His pain was nearly gone and he had energy he hadn't had in years.

6th Key: Never Give Up! Patience and Persistence

Interestingly, the words "patience" *and* "patients" are derived from the same Latin root, *pacient,* which means to suffer or endure. It is no wonder that when we are a patient, we must exercise patience!

Patience is the willingness and strength to wait for the desired results to kick in. Lack of patience makes us restless, scattered, and ultimately impotent to affect changes in our life and our health.

There is an art to practicing patience—a fine line that you learn through experience. If you are overly patient, and trust that something will change when you really need to take action, or if you place too much faith in a treatment that is not working, you may not be driving yourself forward strongly enough. On the other hand, when you are impatient, you're not allowing the time that is needed for something to take effect, so you also won't move forward because you're constantly jumping from one thing to the next. The way to learn the dance between patience and persistence is by practicing, paying attention, and trusting the process. It also involves timing—which is covered in the 3rd Fundamental.

Actions for the 1st Fundamental
The Yin and Yang of Patience and Persistence

1. **Search for Alternative Solutions**
   - Look at what you have done already. If it's not working, what else could you do? What other options are there? Do you need a new practitioner, a new modality?
   - Have a conversation with your caretaker, doctor or healer. Let them know you feel stuck, and that you need help with ideas to move forward.
   - Initiate productive experimenting. Think outside the box (when

the downside is not disastrous). Get online. Widen your perspective.
- Try many things, and then commit to what works!

2. **Go back to the drawing board. Use and explore the first 5 Keys:**
   - Do you feel cared for? Are you focusing on loving your body? How can you bring more love into your daily life? (1st Key)
   - Make sure that your Triangle of Wellness—your immune system, nervous system, and hormones—are in balance. If you are struggling with staying focused and moving forward, you may want to get these checked. (2nd Key)
   - Review your recent lifestyle choices and see if there are any changes that you've made that might be affecting you. What can you do to give your body more support? (3rd Key)
   - Listen. What is your body trying to tell you? Look at your symptoms to find answers. (4th Key)
   - What emotions are you feeling when you feel stuck? Is it anger? Sadness? What can you do to feel better emotionally? (5th Key)

3. **Stop Talking About Your Pain**

   Sometimes, the more you talk about something, the more it's in the forefront of your experience. See what happens to your body when you stop talking about what is bothering you. Try to not complain for a whole day, or a whole week.

4. **Remember, Random Occurrences Aren't Random**

   One thing can lead to the next. You are on a heroic journey. You are healing!

6th Key: Never Give Up! Patience and Persistence

2nd Fundamental
Never Give Up!

ANNE

Anne was 46 when she first came to me for chronic sore throats, laryngitis, and sinus infections. She also had a history of several autoimmune diseases. She explained that she had been consistently ill for the past five years. As a music teacher, Anne's specific illness affected her work and her daily life more than it might affect most people. I asked her in one of our first sessions if she wanted to get well. She told me that she didn't know.

Anne was rather shocked at her own response, and as we explored her feelings, she realized that her illness allowed her to function at a lower capacity and excused her from taking on greater responsibility in her career and life. As she explored her feelings, she realized that feeling better might require her to do more with her time, which felt overwhelming. I told her that the first step to feeling better was committing to her health, and that the process was going to require hard work. Anne decided that she did want feel better.

Once she committed to being healthy, she was persistent. Using a combination of supplements, acupuncture, herbs, and dietary changes, Anne slowly began to experience the results of her commitment. Every time she had a downturn in her health she continued to work on herself—physically, emotionally, and spiritually. She used her physical health as a springboard toward greater emotional and spiritual well-being and implemented each of the 7 Keys.

Within two years of determined focus and practice on her health, Anne was no longer becoming sick. Her autoimmune diseases went into remission. Today, Anne hasn't taken antibiotics in more than ten years.

FLINT TO OUR FIRE

Never give up. These simple words are the standard by which heroes, champions, rock stars, masters, and CEO's live. So many people, both today and historically, have agreed that in order to succeed, *you just keep going.* Knowing that others have gone through their own trials ahead of us can sometimes serve as flint to our fire.

Abraham Lincoln failed at business, and was defeated in eight elections including congress, senate, and even vice president. He then succeeded in becoming one of the most influential presidents in history.

Thomas Edison's teachers told him he was too stupid to learn anything. He was fired from his first two jobs for being unproductive. He made 1,000 failed attempts at inventing the lightbulb. To this he said, *"I didn't fail 1,000 times. The light bulb was an invention with 1,000 steps."*

Oprah Winfrey was fired from her first TV job as an anchor in Baltimore. Walt Disney was fired as a newspaper editor for lack of creativity. Dr. Seuss's first book was rejected by 27 publishers. Michael Jordan was cut from his high school basketball team.

What is the secret ingredient that allows some to keep going, while others give up?

GROWTH MINDSET

> *"Success is not final, failure is not fatal: it is the courage to continue that counts."*
> —WINSTON S. CHURCHILL

Dr. Carol Dweck, a psychology professor at Stanford, has developed a concept called "Growth Mindset." Her hypothesis is that the brain is strengthened by challenges, and that our intelligence is not determined at birth, but can actually be developed.

Dr. Dweck has found that when children learn, the brain *grows* in response to challenges, and that our ability to learn is not fixed but can change with effort, making them more likely to persevere when they fail. When these children make a mistake, they see it as an opportunity to learn and not as a sign of their shortcomings. Therefore, failure is not a permanent condition to them.

Having a "growth mindset" about health, and believing that change is possible, creates more grit and compassion for your process. As my patient Julia discovered (in the beginning of this chapter), *every step is precious and important.* If a treatment does not give you the results you want, it does not mean you wasted your time. It just means that you haven't yet found what you're seeking.

Your healing may not look how you expect—or how you desire. Here is the trick: believe in your tremendous healing ability *and* trust that your healing is happening exactly as it should. At the same time, always continue to seek the healing that you desire.

GRIT

Probably the most important distinction between a person with indomitable grit, and one who gives up, is that the gritty person believes that she can affect the outcome.

Grit has nothing to do with talent, luck, perfection, or genius. Grit is a "never-say-die" attitude. It's about having the drive and gumption to keep your goal in view and to keep moving forward no matter what problems might arise. Grit means having devotion and appreciation for the long haul, and not being sidetracked by hurdles or for your desire for immediate gratification along the way. Gritty people don't fear failure; they see upsets as part of the growing process.

To live with the knowledge that you are truly vulnerable and to keep moving forward toward your goal is an act of great heroism. We can cultivate this never-give-up attitude. And when we do that, we sometimes open the door to the miraculous.

Actions for the 2nd Fundamental
Never Give Up!

1. **The Best Way to Never Give Up? Stay Busy!**
   - Keep busy! Consider Newton's Law of Inertia: an object in motion tends to stay in motion; an object at rest tends to stay at rest. Don't allow lethargy or passivity or despair take over. Continue moving forward, even if your movement feels small or unsure.
   - Set small goals that move you toward your healing. This can be something as simple as taking your medication on time, or exercising, or making sure that you eat green vegetables every day. Each week, make a short list of goals that you can complete. This sense of accomplishment will help increase your motivation.

2. **Make Decisions About Your Healing**
   - Don't wait and put it off.
   - Figure out what you want to change and make it happen!

3. **Patience for the Hard Times**
   Even though so much of the 6th Key is figuring out how to move forward no matter what, it is also important to have patience with yourself for the ups and downs of your journey. When you go through something intensely painful, either physically or emotionally, it can be difficult to stay motivated and moving forward on your path. In those moments, it is OK to not push yourself. In those moments, you don't actually need to *do*

very much, you just need to survive. Focus on what you need to feel OK. Then, once you have moved through that moment, you can pick yourself up again and begin moving forward again.

3rd Fundamental
Divine Timing

Jack

My patient Jack needed hip replacement surgery for about five years. When he first came in to see me, he hobbled in with a cane, in obvious pain. He was a big man, 6-foot-4 and weighing more than 350 pounds. His surgeon wouldn't do the operation until he'd lost 150 pounds. He was scheduled to have the operation in six months, but he had so much pain he needed acupuncture to relieve it and to help him lose weight.

Six months came and went. Jack didn't lose enough weight, and his surgeon refused to do the operation. He would make progress with weight loss and then stop moving forward. Then, Jack got sick and had to go to the hospital for a kidney infection. After he had recovered from that, he had an episode of atrial fibrillation, which put him back in the hospital. The hip replacement operation was postponed over and over. Finally, after four years of trying, Jack lost enough weight and his health was stable enough for the surgery.

Ironically, at that point, his surgeon became ill and had to retire. Jack found another surgeon who had developed a less invasive technique for the hip replacement. This saved Jack from having to go through a huge operation where he would have been in recovery and pain for months.

Less than a month after his surgery, Jack was walking on his new hip. In fact, he almost danced into the office when he came for his follow-ups after the procedure. His personality completely transformed.

Jack went through so much, emotionally, spiritually, and physically in the five years before his surgery. Some of those things we may never fully understand, but he never gave up wanting to be healthy. He came back again and again to fulfill his desire to achieve a more pain-free existence and have a healthier body. The healing that happened, through those years of effort, transformed Jack's life.

To me, Jack is a Hero.

He never gave up. He looked for answers where there didn't seem to be any. He found solutions even though he encountered huge obstacles. And in the end, he was grateful for the ups and downs of his journey, because all of it brought him to a better place than he could have even imagined. All of those qualities are what a hero needs to fulfill his mission.

Timing Is Everything

Patience has never been my strong suit. So much so, that I began my surgical residency because I wanted to fix people *instantaneously!* I understand deeply the struggle of exercising patience. One thing that's helped me feel more patient is realizing that healing requires patience for *everyone* at some point on their journey.

Sometimes you reach a plateau where you are not seeing the same degree of results you saw at the onset of the treatment. The middle part of the healing journey can sometimes be the most difficult. In the beginning, it's exciting. Everything is new, and changing—hopefully for the better. In the middle, when the goal is still distant on the horizon, it can be easy to lose focus, to want to give up, to want to find a faster path. Sometimes, practicing patience and waiting for the opening is the most powerful—and the most difficult—part of the journey.

All too often, when we don't see immediate results, we want to give up. When we fail to give something the time that it needs to work, it is like planting seeds and not watering them, and then just planting more seeds when the first ones don't grow.

6th Key: Never Give Up! Patience and Persistence

Healing does not operate on an imposed timetable. Healing may take a long time, or it can happen in an instant, but healing has its own timing—a perfect timing.

THE FINESSE OF PERFECT TIMING

> *"You don't have to swing hard to hit a home run.*
> *If you got the timing, it'll go."*
> —YOGI BERRA

How do we develop timing? How do we know when it is time to try something new? When is the "right" time?

A baseball player can have an amazing swing, but if the timing is not right, if the ball fails to hit the bat at *just* the right moment, the power of their swing doesn't matter. So how do they learn the art of perfect timing? They practice. Again and again. Beyond their innate skill, their experience gives them their expertise.

Developing a sense of timing does not happen overnight. As we journey, we begin to understand the rhythms of our lives, and how there is a "right time to heal" when everything falls into place. The trick is to take the right actions to make sure your healing happens, and to also trust that there is perfect timing in your healing process.

Actions and Exercises for the 3rd Fundamental Divine Timing

1. **Practice:** Developing timing is about learning the balance between patience and persistence. The Yin essence of patience brings quiet questioning, and patience to hear the answer. The Yang essence of persistence pushes to find the right information, the right doctor, the right medication. Like a baseball player, we can learn to know when to act, when to refrain, and how to follow through. We can learn to sense when something has been played out, when it is time to stop. These timing skills are developed through trial and error, through practice, through paying attention to your body at each step of the process.

2. **Seek guidance:** It can be helpful to seek expert guidance in order to gain a sense of timing. An expert will know when the steps are leading in the right direction or not. Our perceptions and understanding are sometimes not as clear when we are going through something painful or traumatic. Also, during the healing process, you might feel worse before you feel better, or you may not know why you're feeling a certain way, or what you can do to help yourself. Your doctor, or a specialist, can hopefully help you understand what is happening and lead you in the right direction. You can also talk to other patients who are having similar experiences, or find a support group.

3. **Don't be too attached to your plan:** If something is not working, it's wise to recognize that and shift. Sometimes we hold onto something because we've been doing it for so long and we don't want to admit defeat or

failure. Be ready to let go of your idea of how something is going to work, and change depending upon the results and the circumstances. The ability to adapt and be flexible leads to success in all things—including your healing.

4th Fundamental
Believe in Miracles

"There are only two ways to live your life: as though nothing is a miracle, or as though everything is a miracle."
—Albert Einstein

Richard
Richard was diagnosed with incurable stomach cancer. He had recently lost 30 pounds and could no longer eat. The doctors told him not to bother with chemotherapy or surgery, since it would not extend his life and he would just be more physically miserable. They told him he had a month to live.

Richard had a large family, and a large community of friends. Everyone gathered together (for a healing party) to have a long healing conversation in support of Richard. More than 100 people attended, and each person had the opportunity to share their experiences and their love for Richard. He also took this time to talk about the things he felt he was holding onto emotionally, and everyone else did the same. It was a powerful and healing night. Afterward, within one week, Richard was able to eat again. His tumor shrank!

"Do you believe in miracles?" A patient asked me this years ago. Even though I had witnessed and taken part in miraculous healings, like Richard's shrunken tumor, I realized, in that moment, I wasn't sure anymore.

I always had an expectation from life to produce miracles in the way that

I *knew* was possible. Since the day I learned of my great grandmother's death, I had believed in miracles. In my heart, I *knew* that even someone who was very sick, or on their deathbed, could miraculously and instantaneously heal. So, when I looked for a miracle in the life of one of my patients, I envisioned them cured of their disease, healthy and happy, with no further problems. In my experience, that sort of miracle has been rare.

Some of my training as a physician, early on in my career, had me believing that miracles were in my hands. Surgeons really do take people from the brink of death sometimes. Eventually, I came to understand that even though sometimes a life was saved because of my actions, the miracle came from someplace else. Life and death were not in my hands.

As I looked at my patient's expectant face, I realized that I did believe in miracles. It's just that my definition of the miraculous had changed.

Sometimes the miracle is the person in front of us, offering a glimmer of hope or solace, walking beside us on the journey. Sometimes surgery is the miracle, transporting our physical condition from one state to another in a matter of moments or hours, and offering our body an opportunity to reset and heal anew. Sometimes a medication or a healer is a miracle. Sometimes we learn spiritual lessons through our physical experiences—and that can be miraculous.

Chinese medicine taught me to trust that the body knows what it needs to do. Certainly, when we are in pain or in fear, this can be very difficult, in the same way that believing in miracles can be difficult when you have been struggling with something for a long time. But it doesn't mean we should give up. Miracles happen, and they can happen to you. If we live our lives as though everything is a miracle, as if something extraordinary is going to happen, at any moment, life becomes more radiant. Allowing your heart to be open to the miracles in your life, lights the fire of hope.

6th Key: Never Give Up! Patience and Persistence

Actions and Exercises for the 4th Fundamental Believe in Miracles

We usually only think of miracles as these *huge* things that happen. However, if we pay attention to the little, everyday miracles in life, it helps us change our perspective and become more open to the miraculous.

1. **Flowers:** Flowers are so incredibly beautiful and interesting—their variety, their amazing colors, their ephemeral nature. … If you look closely, each one can seem like a miracle! Go for a walk in the botanical gardens, or in nature, or buy yourself some flowers. Their presence is a reminder of an everyday miracle that you can see and touch.

2. **The miracle of life:** Read about how an embryo develops. From the moment of conception, there are millions of things that have to go right in order for a normal human baby to be born. When you learn how much could possibly go wrong, you will look at every life as an absolute miracle.

3. **Miracles in your own life:** Think about all the things that have happened in the last week: can you think of any miracles? There are big miracles, like saving a life, but there are also miracles that seem smaller, but still full of wonder. Every day that you make it safe through freeway traffic, every moment you have with a loved one, when you make a new friend (even if it's a momentary friendship), when you have an amazing meal, the beauty of nature … each of these things is a miracle. What are the miracles in your life?

4. **Alternative news**: Read the news today with miracles in mind. Look for the good stories, the acts of kindness, the willingness to love, the people whose lives were altered in a good way. If you can't find any through normal channels, browse through Facebook to see the good stories. Put a big "Love" on them!

5th Fundamental
Hope

"Hope is the thing with feathers
That perches in the soul
And sings the tune without the words
And never stops—at all."
—EMILY DICKINSON

A LOSS OF HOPE

Richard, my patient and friend with stomach cancer, who received so much love from his community, lived much longer than his doctors had predicted. But even though his tumor had shrunk, and he was able to eat again and felt so much better, the cancer was still present and his doctors' diagnosis was still bleak. They continued to tell him that his cancer was terminal.

Eventually, as the focus was taken off Richard, and people began to turn to their own lives, Richard had to start drawing on his own energy to heal. He did not feel hopeful about his condition. He again began to lose his appetite and lose weight.

At that point, Richard decided that he did not want to fight. He told us that he had decided to quit trying—that he had made a decision to die. He died six weeks later.

6th Key: Never Give Up! Patience and Persistence

From what I have seen, people don't give up when they feel challenged. They give up when they lose hope.

It is very painful, and can be debilitating, to encounter feelings of hopelessness. It might be the most painful part of our journey. The negativity, in our own minds and in the world around us, including the medical world, is a tremendous and arduous hurdle to overcome.

So how do we build our hope, especially when we've been struggling with something for so very long? How can we continue to believe that our condition is going to change, when, despite all our efforts, we still haven't healed? And why should we *want to* build our hope?

For one thing, hope literally benefits your healing—both emotionally and physically. Science shows that hope helps the body heal. When we *believe* that the future is going to bring the results we desire, endorphins are released in the brain, which calms the nervous system in a way that is similar to the effects of morphine.

But it is not enough to just hope for something. In order to progress, it means believing that there are possibilities for healing, and taking action toward what gives you hope. If you don't *believe* that you are going to heal, your efforts are more like "going through the motions," and therefore not as effective. It's the difference between wishing you felt better, and using all of your resources to take action and move toward your hope and your healing.

Hope is such a rich experience. It is worth the effort to build it, to focus on it, to recognize that it is the spark that can light your own inner fire. Hope is what keeps us going, even in the dark, even when things seem impossible. Eagerly and expectant, we hope for the things yet to come, for our dreams to be our reality, for possibility. Everything relies on hope.

Actions and Exercises for the 5th Fundamental Hope

1. **Build Your Hope**
    - The nature of hope is to seek something you don't already have. That is why, on your healing path, it is important to set many goals and to have many hopes. Once you have achieved one thing, set another goal. This keeps you moving forward.
    - Hope can be triggered, but not forced. Wherever you feel hope, go there and focus on that. If you've been told a story that feels hopeless, look for something that makes you feel hopeful.
    - Go to a practitioner who believes in your healing. Surround yourself with people who are supportive of your healing journey. If you are having trouble claiming your power and believing in yourself, get a friend or support person to advocate for you. There are times on the journey where we need assistance to get back to those places of hope.
    - A quality of hope is believing you have the power to make your hopes your reality. Explore what is going to make you feel powerful. Maybe it's your faith in a higher power. Maybe it's your love for your children or family. Maybe it's your belief in your own strength and destiny. Whatever it is, build on that.
    - Remember that you are not just your illness or your pain. Make sure that you maintain your identity outside of your illness. Identify with your children, your career, your creativity, your passions. Look at yourself and ask, "Where and who am I in this process?"
    - When illness seems purposeless, it feels hopeless. Find a purpose that makes sense to *you*.

Chapter 7

7th Key: Trusting the Process

"What the caterpillar calls the end of the world, the master calls a butterfly."
—RICHARD BACH

MICHAEL

I met Michael when he was 39. He had just been diagnosed with terminal cancer and was having trouble breathing. The cancer was in his pleurae, which is the fluid-filled layer of tissue that surrounds the lungs. In Michael, this fluid was filled with cancer cells, which were compressing his lungs and making it difficult to breathe.

His doctors did not know where the cancer originated, so they felt they could not aggressively treat it with chemo or radiation. They told him there was no hope of recovery and said that he would not live past April 1. It was September when we met. Michael and I were the same age.

Even though his doctors told him that his cancer was incurable, Michael was still looking for hope, which is why he came to see me. His presence in my life had an immeasurable impact.

I became deeply invested in trying to save Michael's life. Since we were the same age it felt especially poignant that he was facing death, and that his doctors had not given him any options. I did not believe that he should be "condemned" to death and I felt that I could do something about it. I had witnessed miracles, and I was determined that together we could save his life.

Michael came to see me every week. He was open and receptive to my ideas, and we tried everything: diet, acupuncture, herbs, supplements. He explored and tried to understand his emotional traumas. He even had one round of chemo—but it didn't change anything. None of our efforts seemed to have an impact. I watched, feeling helpless, as his health deteriorated. There was a sense that his fate was already determined.

Michael greatly appreciated all my efforts. He told me that our work together helped him connect to his loved ones, so that he was able to express himself and have more closure. In the last few months, Michael made peace with his loved ones. He focused on what was really important to him, and shared with his family and friends how he felt. His wife and family were grateful for the changes that happened and the healing that occurred in those last months of his life.

On March 31, Michael became short of breath early in the morning. He died before the ambulance arrived.

Letting Go

When Michael died, I was devastated. I took his death personally. At that time in my life, I felt that I should have been able to save someone like Michael. I had invested every ounce of my faith and abilities into trying to heal him, and in the end, it seemed like I had failed him.

If someone had told me to "trust the process" as Michael was dying, I probably would have wanted to throw something at them.

Finding trust, especially when life is not giving us what we want, feels like an impossible task. It almost seems pointless. Why trust, when it's not going to change the outcome? Why trust, when nothing is guaranteed? Why trust, when bad things happen, and no amount of trust can take away the pain of those moments?

I thought that through my knowledge and through the force of my will I could make a miracle happen. But I was not in control, and Michael's death uprooted my trust. I was fighting so hard to make him better that I couldn't see Michael's death offered a beautiful healing for both Michael and his family. At that time, all I saw was loss.

After Michael died, I had to let go of so many beliefs that had driven me as a doctor and a healer. I didn't want to let them go—they had been the source of my resolve and strength for my whole life. But I was torturing myself, thinking that I had failed, thinking that it was somehow my fault, feeling angry at life and at God for not allowing Michael to live.

Life sometimes pushes us into experiencing the opposite of what we want—the opposite of our hopes and dreams. My devastation after Michael's death forced me to let go of my ideas of what I thought needed to happen, and allowed me to open up to something bigger, something mysterious and unseen.

Eventually, I realized that while I could soothe, guide, encourage, and support someone on their healing journey, and I could diagnose and treat them, the actual healing comes from a deeper place. This revelation was incredibly humbling, but also incredibly powerful in my work. I began to trust and give room for each person's process. I stopped feeling responsible for the things that were beyond my control. These gentle shifts made me more open to the divine, and more available to listen to the desires and needs of my patients.

Trusting the process doesn't mean that you're always going to receive what you want. It doesn't mean that you can control everything. Trusting the process means that you believe in your healing—no matter what. It means that you trust the right things are happening, and that you are taking the steps you need to take. It means that you are open to something greater than you.

Healing When It Seems Impossible

ACCELERATED HEALING

I've mentioned this story before, but it serves here again as an example: Years ago I had a knee problem that made it painful to walk and dance. At the time, I wanted to lose about 20 pounds, and I was using exercise and diet to do it. My knee problem made exercise difficult, but I had the hardest time giving it up!

Finally, the pain was so bad that I was forced to let my leg rest. I began doing more gentle exercises like Qi Gong and yoga, and I actually lost the 20 pounds faster than when I was trying so hard! I worked with my knee to learn what was best for it, and in the end, it was better for both my weight goal and my knee.

It may seem counterintuitive to relax and let your body guide you, especially when you are having pain and your body is acting up. When you are in pain, it can feel like your body is just screaming at you. Sometimes, relaxing, slowing down, or letting go is exactly what your body needs to heal.

When we feel ill, we never want to let it take over. We resist it with all our might. We want to figure out what's wrong and tackle the problem, but in my experience, that rarely creates the healing we want. I've learned that healing is actually faster when you surrender to the process and treat your body with love, accepting that you are learning something. Of course, you always try to find out what is wrong and work to heal it, you just let go of the intensity of the struggle.

The idea is that when we resist something, it slows down. The very nature of resistance is to oppose the force of something. Sometimes by trying so hard to change our experience, we actually end up slowing down the healing process. By working *with* the forces you feel are against you, as I did with my knee, you can actually speed up the healing process and create what I call Accelerated Healing.

When you feel more relaxed, you can find a way to tap into what your body is trying to say and find solutions more quickly. The gift of Accelerated

Healing is that it allows you to *immediately* move into a place of wholeness and well-being, simply by dropping the fight.

Very often, when I try so hard to move forward, the effort seems to stop me from moving forward. My body is often what forces me to slow down and take it easy. Having an issue that doesn't get better forces me to look at it from every angle, and this process always brings me greater overall health.

What Do You Do When You Don't Have Control?

"Everything can be taken from a man but one thing: the last of the human freedoms—to choose one's attitude in any given set of circumstances, to choose one's own way."
—Viktor E. Frankl

Until now, this book has focused on how you can have more control over your body, and ways you can prevent illness, create more balance, and maintain your health. But what about when something happens that is truly beyond your control? What about when you are confronted with the unbearable and you can't find relief?

Certain events happen in life—and we have no choice. If you're in a fire or a hurricane, you don't have a choice. None of us have a choice about aging. And pain is often something where we have very little control. Even pain medication cannot touch some super painful places.

Pain, fear, and trauma can take us away from who we are. We can forget our purpose, our strength, our drive. We lose touch with what makes us happy. We lose faith, and it's like the rug has been pulled out from under us. How do you find your feet again when this happens? How do you build your faith when your experiences seem to be telling you that whatever you're doing is not working? And when you are shrouded in fear and doubt, how do you find the light, the trust, the faith, again?

This is exactly where the 7th Key can help.

The idea of *trusting the process* when you are in that place might seem like an inane solution to a humongous problem. It might make you angry. I know that's how I feel at times. *But*, what I have witnessed and experienced in my own life and body, and from what I have seen in my patients, is that when you don't trust, your ability to heal is impacted. When you don't trust, you stop being able to hear to your own intuition. You stop believing that you are meeting the right people and taking the right actions. Your confidence is replaced by self-doubt and insecurity. When you don't have trust and you are in pain or having a serious issue with your body, it's like falling off a cliff into darkness.

The 7th Key helps us find our faith when we've lost it. It allows us to take the next step forward, even when we don't know what's going to happen. And, it allows us to open up to possibilities that may be beyond our understanding.

After so many years of working with people and helping patients and loved ones go through extraordinarily difficult and painful moments, I am still hopeful. I have learned something very important: There is an innate healing that exists within each of us, and it is happening all the time. With this understanding, there is no blame for your body or your experiences. Everything has the potential to heal, to inspire growth, and to transform.

Working with Alchemy

The 7th Key works like alchemy. Alchemy is an ancient science, religion, and philosophy that has been practiced all around the world for more than 4,000 years. It is founded on the belief that base metals like lead, tin, copper, or nickel can be transmuted into gold through a mystical process. The 7th Key allows us work with alchemy in our own bodies. When we learn to trust the process, we are taking something that is ordinary or difficult in regard to our health, and turning it into something profound and transcendent. We all have the ability to transform our experiences so that they give us energy, feed us, and help us grow.

This simple, instantaneous, alchemic transformation happens when we can *recognize and trust the spiritual (or energetic) connection that we have to our bodies.* The body, like the universe, is mysterious. Instead of feeling overwhelmed or frightened by the unknown, why not feel empowered by the potential magic that exists within you? When we do this, our perspective shifts toward our healing.

Trusting the process is not passive, even though it might sound as though it is. It is an action. It is a decision, just like maintaining a healthy lifestyle. It requires attention. If you are fighting your circumstances, or angry and feeling betrayed, or wanting to put your head in the sand, all of your energy is going toward that fight rather than toward your healing. When you trust what is happening, there is a greater flow, greater movement, and greater possibility in your experiences.

It's no accident that the 7th Key is the final Key. Trusting the process of life is deep inner work. The willingness to put one foot in front of the other when everything is uncertain and painful requires incredible courage, stamina, strength, flexibility, and drive. All of the work that you've done with the other 6 Keys is going to help you when you don't feel in control, and when healing seems impossible.

> ## Fundamentals of the 7th Key
>
> Throughout this book I have explained that fundamentally, healing takes time—*the quick fix is not necessarily the best fix.* There is one caveat to that rule: the 7th Key can happen in an instant and it can be used every day, in any situation and at any moment. It is simultaneously the most simple, the most immediate, and the most ethereal of all the 7 Keys.
>
> The 7th Key is a guide to find what works for *you*, rather than step-by-step instructions. Remember, you are working with alchemy and the 7th Key is like a magic elixir. Trusting the process can be attained instantaneously, and it can influence each element of your health fully and potently.

1st Fundamental: Dealing with Pain
Being alive means experiencing times of suffering and pain. We each have to learn to live with this, process through the pain, and find a way to be OK—no matter what might be happening in our lives. Trusting the process when we are in pain can feel infuriating, excruciating, and unfair, but once we get past our resistance, there are immeasurable benefits—not only to our healing, but also to our experience of pain.

2nd Fundamental: From Fear to Faith
Why is faith so important on your healing journey? What does it mean for you to have faith? It does not have to mean something religious, but to believe in your healing, and to have faith that you are healing *at this very moment,* is incredibly helpful to the healing process.

3rd Fundamental: Acceptance and Surrender

To be alive, and to know and accept that you are truly vulnerable, and to find a way to be OK with that and with everything that happens to your body, is the spiritual aspect of your physical healing. Acceptance and surrender allow you to witness your pain and vulnerability, and actually gain strength from them.

4th Fundamental: Seeing the Big Picture

Your spirit affects your life and your health. You are intricately a part of the world, and there is a flow to the life and energy that is happening all around you. Recognizing this—that your spiritual well-being affects your body, and that it stems from your connection to the greater universe—is an important aspect of the 7th Key.

1st Fundamental
Dealing with Pain

*"Pain is important: how we evade it, how we succumb to it,
how we deal with it, how we transcend it."*
—AUDRE LORDE

CAN YOU TRUST YOUR BODY WHEN IT HURTS?

Imagine one morning you wake up with a sudden severe pain in your back. You can hardly straighten your body and you feel like if you breathe you're going to fall over. Every step is pure agony. There's nothing that makes it feel better. You go to the ER and they take X-rays and give you a shot to reduce the pain, but that only holds for a little while. Worst of all, they can't find anything wrong with you.

Over several weeks you are gradually able to straighten your body, but the pain is still there. You can't find anyone who can solve the problem for you, and now it's impeding your activities—so you're annoyed. After another month, you go from being annoyed to being afraid that there's something seriously wrong with you. And even though every doctor and specialist is telling you that there's nothing wrong, you are still in pain, and you have this insistent feeling that something's not right.

What do you do when you are in pain? Do you try to understand it, or do you just try to find relief and make it go away? If the pain continues, can you find a way to still trust your body?

I never want anyone to be in pain. Even though I firmly trust the body's process, I always put every effort into taking away someone's pain. This may sound like a contradiction—trust your body, even when it's in pain, *and* do everything in your power to make the pain go away—but it's an important part of the healing process.

Think of your body as an antenna. It's always speaking to you—giving and receiving information. When you are ill or in pain, try to see what is happening to you as a communication, instead of believing that your body is breaking down and needs to be fixed. Being trusting creates the potential for you to interact with your body and to learn from it. Being trusting naturally gives your experiences value and meaning.

This doesn't mean that you *want* to be sick or injured. You would never choose it. But there is a way to figure out how to leverage your experience so you can gain the most from it and heal at the same time.

Your body is malleable. It wants to heal, and results can happen fast. Trust that your body is speaking to you and trying to tell you something important. It is easier to grow when you are trusting.

Time and again I have seen my patients change their lives when they go through an intense physical issue. When your body acts up, it can be a call to connect to something deeper. Learn from your body and find out: What foods can you eat? What supplements you can take? How much sleep you need? Are there other things you can do to strengthen your body and feel better? What is it that *you* need to feel OK?

There is collaboration at work inside of you. Your body, your mind, your heart, and your spirit—every part of you is working together, building, growing, and creating the person who you are. Just because you are sick doesn't take away the fact that your existence is important and miraculous.

Ben

My patient Ben was 43 years old when his back went out suddenly. It was terrifying. He could not move, or lift, or be in life in any of the ways that he had previously. After weeks of struggling, he started to really pay attention to what was happening to his body. One day he noticed that when he sat a certain way, his back didn't hurt so much. He began to notice that if he didn't eat sugar, his back would hurt less. Slowly, over the course of several months, he began to feel better and notice the things that helped.

Movements, supplements, treatments, and even his mood affected his pain. It was as though his body was showing him a whole new way of living. By using his pain as a guide, and not just something to fix, Ben was able to better understand his body's sensitivities and needs and eventually find relief.

Seeking Safety

Pain tells us when we need to protect ourselves. It tells us not to touch fire, not to walk on an injured ankle, and it helps us know when we need to seek medical help. It is much more complex than a simple neurological response. In order to feel pain from a cut on your finger, your body has to communicate with your brain, and your brain has to tell you that it hurts. Part of the brain's assessment is the degree of danger, or the potential risk, of the experience.

Studies have shown that if your brain perceives that the danger is great, your experience of pain will be more intense. During World War II, it was found that soldiers who were hospitalized for their injuries suffered much less pain than was normal, because they were no longer on the battlefield. They felt safe, so this reduced their sense of pain.

When you feel threatened, your experience of pain tends to be heightened. This means that when the reason for your pain is unknown, or the prognosis is unclear, it is not only terribly frightening, it can also actually be more painful due to that uncertainty.

It's important to note that even though our experience of pain comes from the brain, it does not mean we can mentally control pain—it's much more instinctual than that. We can, though, work on finding ways to feel more safe and secure when we are in pain. Remember, pleasure feels good, and it also feels *safe*. Knowing that your pain actually might be reduced if you find ways to feel safe can be a strong motivator. Try to build those relationships and dynamics that make you feel supported. Focus on what makes you feel good, and see how that changes your experience.

Why Pain?

Asking ourselves *"Why?"* when we are in pain can turn up some pretty terrible answers. We don't ask *"Why is this happening to me?"* from a place of power, and our stance on this healing path is the stance of a Hero—valiant and taking charge. Still, when we are confronted with extreme or continuous pain, our minds can't help but ask *why*. Thankfully, there are actually some very good answers.

Although we may never understand exactly why we experience particular difficulties in our lives, we all know that pain can initiate transformation. Something happens to people when they go through pain *that is positive*. As Aristotle stated, *"We cannot learn without pain."* Oftentimes, something in our lives has to break down in order for us to change it.

Heroes go through extreme physical pain in order to reach their goal. A "trial by fire" strengthens them, demonstrates their bravery, and proves that they are able to perform under pressure. This same philosophy is true with surgeons, police officers, firefighters, people in the military, and anyone who is an apprentice of an art or a practice. It seems that intensive training is a part of proving our fortitude and commitment in these challenging careers.

Pain is also a motivator. It can help us learn; *"no pain, no gain!"* We "feel the burn" at the gym. We are excited by challenges at work.

Our emotional discomfort can sometimes force us to take leaps and change in ways we wouldn't have dreamed. We appreciate all of these moments because we're moving toward a goal, and we're making the choice to do it.

It's different, though, when the reason for our pain is unknown, or relentless, or severe. This kind of pain is what often shows up in the body, and when that happens, it's simply awful. It doesn't feel like anything good can come from it.

I have a friend who recently went through an excruciating experience after surgery. The pain medication she was given didn't help, and it made her feel dizzy and sick, so she quit taking it. The only thing that helped was acupuncture.

When she began to feel better, I asked her how she got through it, and she said she focused on incremental improvements. She said that she reminded herself that this, as with everything, was temporary. She told herself: "Get to the next day, the next moment. You're breathing. At least you're breathing. You've got your mind. …" Then, the next day, and the next, she would see and feel small things that showed her she was healing. She chose to focus on those things, and trust them, until one day she began to feel better.

Remember, if your pain takes over, there is only one thing you need to do and that is *survive*. Don't worry about thinking positively, or finding love or meaning, or even trying to *do* anything. All you need to do is figure out how you're going take your next breath.

We attend to our pain because we have to—there's no other way out.

Intense pain and intense pleasure have the ability to bring us into the present moment more than any other experience. To endure pain, and to not give up, and to keep going, and to trust that it will someday get better, requires the greatest strength inside a person.

It's like the making of a crucible. In order to create a vessel that can withstand the heat of liquid gold and metal, clay and sand go through a transformational process. Prolonged, extreme heat gives ordinary substances superhero strength. Through the fire, something altogether new is born.

We can't always find answers to *"why"*. What we *do* know is that when we go through something painful and arrive on the other side, something inside of us has changed. The courage to start that journey—even if it's completely forced upon us—to put one foot in front of the other, with our eyes on the horizon, and on the hope for light, is brave, and heroic, and incredibly human.

Actions for the 1st Fundamental Dealing with Pain

Remember, if your pain takes over, don't worry about *doing* anything. Trying to do more when you are experiencing overwhelming pain can just create more struggle, more pain. All you need to do is survive it—and that is heroic.

1. **Ease Your Nervous System**

    Healing isn't always about making your pain go away, it's also about finding a way to be OK when you are in pain. Often, pain is an overwhelming sensation that seems to grow out of the location in your body where it started, and it takes over. If you are dealing with pain, try to do everything you can to ease your nervous system.

- Do things that give you pleasure. Feed yourself food that is nurturing. Take a hot bath. Move your body in ways that feel good. You may even try pushing against the places that feel pain—and show your body that it can move, that it is healing.
- Quiet your body down. Take some deep breaths and begin to listen to the places you feel the pain. Keep breathing and listening. Follow the sensations with your mind, and just observe. If something is particularly painful, search for a position that will ease the discomfort. Do this with a sense of curiosity—*i.e.,* if your knee hurts, try straightening your leg to see if it lessens the pain. Then try bending it in a different way. Make your movements gentle and patient. Keep breathing deeply and listening to the sensations you have. Do this for at least two minutes a day.
- Another nervous system calming action is to gently stroke your skin. This can be anyplace, but if nothing else, stroke your arms up and down. Do this with a very light touch, like a feather. You can do it along your legs, and belly or wherever it is easy for you to reach. Light butterfly touches relax your nervous system.

2. **Asking the Right Questions**

    When you are focused on the wrong question (like, "Why is this happening to me?") you don't get the answers that will open doors for healing. Instead of thinking of all the things that aren't working, or feeling bad about what you can't do, ask: "What do I need right now?" "What is my next step?" "Is there something I can say or do that will make it better?"

2nd Fundamental
From Fear to Faith

Emma

Emma has been my patient for almost 20 years. She started seeing me in her 60's and is now 87. Lately, she has been having more and more difficulty with her body. She is nauseated, tired, shaky, and dizzy all the time. In the past two years she has lost 20 pounds. When she comes in, she looks unwell, as if the weight loss is due to illness rather than good health.

She has seen at least 20 doctors since her symptoms began, trying to get to the root cause of it. No one has been able to accurately diagnose her condition. They have given her many medications, none of which have helped. The only thing that seems to make her temporarily better is acupuncture. So, I see Emma once every two weeks for acupuncture. She is one of the kindest people I've met in my career, and is always ready to help someone else in need.

Emma has been a devout orthodox Christian her whole life. One day I asked her about her faith, in relationship to what she was experiencing in her body. She said that she talks to God every day, many times. She said she was told to have patience. She trusts her god, and even though she doesn't understand fully what is happening, she keeps her faith, and trusts that she will heal, and that it is just taking time.

As we talked, Emma became more peaceful and relaxed. We both realized we had to trust her process. Even though she is struggling, she is connecting to her higher purpose through her spiritual faith.

The Paradox

Why is it so hard to trust what we are experiencing physically?

We value challenges at work because they motivate us to find solutions, and we know we become more skilled when we push our limits. When we

7th Key: Trusting the Process

have conflict in our relationships, we can learn about each other and become closer. In the same way, when intense things happen to us physically, we are *meant* to find our way through it. Challenges help us grow and heal, which means that physical issues can also catalyze transformation.

Imagine if, like Emma, you believed wholeheartedly in your ability to heal? Imagine if you had a true sense that your body is working toward your benefit in everything that it does, whatever your age or condition?

For most of my life, I had an inner voice that I trusted completely. It was what guided me to want to be a doctor when I was five years old, to go into surgery residency after I saved a life for the first time, and to study acupuncture when I realized that surgery was not my path. I have complete faith in that voice. When I "hear" it, I listen.

When I was going through my divorce, it seemed that my inner voice went away. I felt rudderless and terrified of what was next. I started to not trust my own internal guidance, and found myself seeking outside validation. I was in a constant state of uncertainty and fear. I not only lost my faith, but the idea of finding faith again seemed absolutely impossible.

When we are in the middle of something, it can be hard to have perspective, to believe that it will ever change. When we can't see the horizon, how do we have faith that it will ever come? Truly, in life, there are very few guarantees, but just because we experience one side of something, doesn't mean that the other side is gone. Just because we are sick, doesn't mean that we won't heal. Just because we experience incredible sadness, doesn't mean that happiness isn't right around the corner.

Life is full of paradoxes: the good and the bad, the pain and the ecstasy, the hope and the despair, the fear and the faith. The truth is, when we are sick, our healing is right there, too. Both exist simultaneously—like Yin and Yang. To be alive means that we will experience both sides throughout our lives. Ultimately, we feel better when we realize this, and find a way to work with this tenuous balance.

I have worked hard on my faith. It seems to me that faith is something that is alive. It grows as we do. When we are afraid, it is simply a calling to go deeper to find our faith and our love.

Our struggles, and loss of faith, can actually be the very things that strengthen us, because when we can't see the light, it is our desire and drive to keep trying, to keep searching, and to stay focused on what is possible that builds our faith. If we were never tested, how would we ever know if our faith was real?

When you lose faith, you don't give up—because your faith is not actually really gone. It's right there, like a seed in the ground in the wintertime. You might not always be able to see it, but those moments when you feel lost are *always* the beginning of something new. Explore your thoughts. Nurture your body. Weed out self-doubt and criticism. Harvest the goodness in your life. Eventually, your faith will surface again, like a flower in the springtime.

Saul

My friend Saul was diagnosed with kidney cancer at age 60. He was told the cancer was incurable, but he didn't give up. I've always admired Saul for his unwavering positive attitude—he sees the good in every situation.

When Saul received the diagnosis, he immediately turned himself over to prayer. He's a deeply religious man, and his friends and family prayed for him, too. Saul found comfort in his faith, and at the same time, he and his wife searched unyieldingly for something that might help him.

They found a clinical trial that Saul's doctors approved. Even though his prognosis was dire, they thought there was a chance it could help. Saul went through the process of having all the tests required for the trial and was approved and ready to begin.

The day that he was scheduled to start, the doctors at the trial told him that, in fact, he would not be able to participate. Stunned, Saul asked them why. They said he did not meet their standards. Apparently, his tumor had shrunk

7th Key: Trusting the Process

and was no longer big enough for them to treat.

Saul believes that through prayer, and through surrendering his life to God, something miraculous happened. He survived the cancer, and is living a healthy, full life to this day.

Faith is incredibly individual. Even within the same spiritual family, people think about things differently. We hold our beliefs close to our hearts—but these quiet, private thoughts impact us on every level, including in our bodies.

Faith is believing in something that you cannot see. One of the reasons that we have faith, and persevere in our search for faith, is that it brings us comfort. Faith makes us feel better, and in life, feeling better is really, really, important. Yes, we want the truth, we don't want to be in denial, but there is so much mystery in the world and in our own bodies. Your choice is to either have faith that you are healing, and to trust—beyond what you can see—or not.

In the end, your faith, and trust, and hope are not something that anyone can give to you. It must be born within you. Your doctors, your healers, your spiritual counselors, your friends, your guides—they can help you tremendously and take you to the very edge of what is possible, but you are the one who must take the final step. You must believe what is right for you. It rests upon your shoulders. It is up to you.

Actions for the 2nd Fundamental
From Fear to Faith

1. **Focus on What Is Working**

    If you are busy wondering why, or beating yourself up for something that you may have done that caused your condition, or hating God, or looking for somewhere to place blame—those thoughts suck your energy and do not bring relief. Focus on what is working, on what is possible. It is a decision, but it is as natural as breathing.

2. **Test Your Faith**

    The best way to build your faith is to test it. When you live as if the worst thing is going to happen at any moment, there is a tendency to make your life smaller. I used to be afraid to do new things, so I began to build my faith by doing small things that scared me.

    You can start by doing something small. Let's say that you are afraid to go out by yourself, and you don't have anyone to go out with. Try going shopping by yourself; that's usually easy to do. Then, go have a cup of coffee alone, in a coffee shop. Again, not too difficult, but it will increase your courage. Then, go to breakfast by yourself. Slowly, you can begin to do more and more things alone, and you will probably notice that you are not so afraid. Maybe you'll even meet some new friends by doing it.

3. **Check the Facts**

    This was an exercise I introduced in the 1st Key (Love), and it is equally important to do now, with the 7th Key.

    Often when we don't have faith, we actually have faith that something bad will happen. Sometimes we live entirely in our heads and don't check the facts. Ask yourself if what you are thinking is really true.

Let's say you are about to go meet your mom for lunch. She always criticizes how you dress. Think about all the times she's done that—has it really been *every* time you meet her for lunch? Even if there's *one* time that she didn't, maybe you can let yourself have faith in a different outcome.

Many of my patients forget their symptoms after they've gone away. As they evolve in their healing, they sometimes develop new symptoms, or *some* of the old ones don't go away. They will say, "I'm not any better." At that point, I go through a checklist of symptoms and ask them to think about each one. Usually, they find that many of the symptoms they had in the beginning have gone away!

Checking the facts is a simple way to reinstate faith in your process.

3rd Fundamental
Acceptance and Surrender

KEN

Once, while I was hiking in Waimea canyon in Kauai, I met a man who was diabetic. We started talking and he told me that he was a brittle diabetic, which is a particularly severe form of diabetes. It meant that he had to monitor his blood sugar all the time because it could easily swing to extremes. He carried his insulin shots with him wherever he went and checked his blood sugar about five times a day. When he was physically active, he knew he'd use up his insulin faster and was able to stay in touch with how he felt so he didn't allow his blood sugar to get too low.

I found out his name was Ken, and when he was a young man, he had tried to ignore that he had diabetes and ended up in the hospital in diabetic shock several times. Once, he almost died. That's when he decided that he could no longer ignore that he had diabetes. Through extensively researching his condition, (this was before the Internet) he learned that he could micromanage his blood sugar and have more control of his life. He also learned that he would be less likely to have kidney failure and loss of his eyesight if he maintained his blood sugar more evenly.

Through accepting that he had this illness, he learned to live with it as a presence in his life. He said that he felt it actually allowed him to have a more active, normal life—because he was paying close attention to his health-care maintenance.

Acceptance

Can you accept your life, exactly as it is, right now?

You might think, "Why would I ever want to accept something that is unacceptable?" A life-threatening or life-changing diagnosis, unexplained or unrelenting physical pain, or any condition that eludes diagnosis makes us want to fight—relentlessly. You might think, "No, I can't accept this." The problem is, in some situations, we become stuck and unable to move forward if we don't stop fighting—like a body in quicksand.

Sometimes the bravest and smartest thing you can do is to stop resisting and accept your experience. Acceptance is *not* giving up or giving in. Acceptance is the willingness to work with what you've got. It is the strength to not condemn your experience, and it requires the grace and resilience of a Hero.

Acceptance says: *This is who I am. This is what I have. Certain things may never change. I accept that, for now, this is the way it is.* This is hard to do, but once you have accepted where you are, you can begin to move forward. You can take the next step, and ask the next question: *What am I going to do NOW?*

Most likely you don't want to accept it. I know that the idea of accepting something painful and unjust is agonizing in itself. But you won't get answers or new ideas when you are sitting in "I hate where I am."

7th Key: Trusting the Process

This is about healing when it seems impossible, and with impossible issues, normal steps don't work. You've already tried that. You wouldn't be here if it were easy. You're here, reading this book, because you're looking for another answer. You want an *inner revolution*.

In all great hero stories, there is a moment when the hero confronts the possibility of his own death. Joseph Campbell calls this the "Supreme Ordeal"—the moment when the hero faces his greatest foe or his greatest fear. Everything that he has learned is put to the test, and he knows he may not survive. That moment, when he conquers his greatest fear, is when the apprentice becomes the master.

For many, the idea of accepting your condition, as it is, right now, is the Supreme Ordeal. *Can you accept your life, exactly as it is, right now?*

Amber

Amber was diagnosed with stage 4 lymphatic cancer when she was 35 years old. When she received her diagnosis, her first thought was that she could "check out." She had recently been divorced and was feeling tired and stuck in her life. But immediately following that thought, she had a deep recognition that the diagnosis was not a death sentence, but an opportunity to transform her life.

The next year of her life was devoted to her healing. She learned to listen to her own body. She was a bodyworker (massage practitioner) by trade, so she was already familiar with being intuitive and the importance of taking care of herself, but her cancer upped the ante of her healing abilities.

The seriousness of her condition thrust her into an immediate state of action and acceptance. She was able to endure the pain of the procedures, the bone biopsies and the chemo with surrender, which she felt ultimately eased the pain. She changed her diet, quit smoking, did chemotherapy, sound healing, and meditation—and eventually, she had a full recovery.

Amber feels that her experience with cancer was a gift, one that enhanced her healing abilities, her compassion, her strength and her ability to connect to her own body. Accepting her condition and surrendering to life and God gave her peace and confidence throughout her healing journey. While she worked on healing from every possible angle, she also knew that it was not completely in her hands. This feeling—of being in God's hands—brought her comfort.

Today, her continued gratitude for her experiences allows her to stay open, and not back away or shut down when life is overwhelming or frightening.

THE POWER OF SURRENDER

"Surrender is the doorway to unlimited strength.
Surrender is the only way to be in a position of power.
Surrender is actively moving forward with no attachment to the results.
Surrender is the ability to change directions at a moment's notice when necessary.
Surrender is stopping the fight. The external fight. The internal fight.
Imagine if you no longer saw yourself as being attacked and having to protect yourself! Suddenly you would not have to use all of your energy to stay safe, you could now use all of your power to solve whatever problem is presenting itself."
—SIVAN GARR

Surrender is different than acceptance. Acceptance is acknowledging where you are: "I accept that I am here. I accept that I have cancer." Surrender is feeling that something greater is in charge: "I surrender my anger. I surrender my pain. I surrender my fear." Surrender is allowing yourself to be cradled by something greater than yourself.

People often think that surrender means you're giving up. For our purposes, and when it comes to your health, surrender is about *opening* yourself up. It is not a sign of weakness or denial, and it is not a failure. Surrender is releasing your demands upon life and allowing something bigger to carry you.

Imagine you are swimming in the ocean and pulled out by a riptide. Some say that the best thing to do is to relax and go with the flow of the water, because if you fight it, you can exhaust yourself and drown. Riptides generally only last about 20-30 meters, so if you ride it out, you'll save your energy and be able swim back to shore once it's run its course. If you fight the tide, you are using precious energy and trying to go someplace the water won't let you go.

The ocean is stronger than you. If your energy is not pushing against the tide of your life, then you have energy to spare for other things—like your healing.

OPENING TO LIFE

When your pet is sick, it doesn't argue with the fact that it feels ill, it just surrenders to the illness and accepts it. There is only the here and now with your dog or cat. It isn't thinking about how it wants to go back to how it used to feel.

Without surrender, we are either holding onto something from the past—the way things used to be—or we are insisting that our experiences be different. Our desire to control gets in the way of our experience of life. Surrender is letting go of what we think life should be like, and opening up to what life has in store for us.

Imagine a closed fist. You can't really hold hands if your fist is closed. You can't receive a gift. You can't eat, or swim, or really do anything! Trying to control everything in your life is like living life with closed fists. Instead, unwind your need to control. Open your hands and be willing to receive what life brings. You might be surprised by what comes.

I know that it is not easy to surrender. There are things in my life I've wanted that have not happened. I've struggled with my own physical pain, with growing older, with the morning traffic. I've struggled watching some of my patients on their own paths. I want every person to feel better, and sometimes things don't change in the way that we want. We can't always be in control.

In those moments when you feel completely helpless and without power, say to yourself: "I surrender this problem to you, the higher ups, so that you can help me with it. I give this to the higher powers—because this is bigger than me." You may find that you have an answer you didn't have before. You may find a bit of ease in your heart. Sometimes, a miracle can happen.

Surrender does not mean you quit trying to make a difference; it means you allow yourself to be where you are. It brings relaxation because you stop putting your energy into places where your efforts are not working. It lowers cortisol. When you relax and rest, other answers can come. Surrender puts you right here, right now, and it gives you space to create, to be new, and to find other solutions.

We don't always see the ways we are protected, the little gifts, when everything lines up despite all our fighting. The divine takes care of us on some level, and our bodies are guiding us to change in ways we have never imagined. This chapter is about trusting the process. Try, for a whole day, trusting that God or Life or a divine energy is right there with you, supporting you in every moment.

Actions for the 3rd Fundamental Acceptance and Surrender

1. **The Worst-Case Scenario Exercise**
   Imagine that your greatest fear comes to pass. This happened to me many years ago when my therapist suggested that I take a month off from my surgical residency. I was so scared that it would cause me to lose my position in the program because there was so much competition around it. My therapist asked me to imagine the worst-case scenario. Of course, my first thought was that I'd be fired. Then she asked me to imagine what would happen if I was fired. I realized that my life would be OK if that happened.

   Think about your health challenge, and imagine that the symptoms you have now will never change. Imagine they even get worse. Take yourself through a life where you will have these symptoms ongoing. What would you do? How would you live? How would you make your life work?

2. **Be Flexible**
   When you do this exercise, you will find a flexibility inside of yourself that will allow you to open up to new solutions. Initially you might feel hopeless, but after you really think about it, you will see new possibilities for healing that you never saw before. This can only happen if you come to a certain acceptance of where you are now.

4th Fundamental
Seeing the Big Picture

"The cure of many diseases is unknown to physicians because they are ignorant of the whole. For the part can never be well unless the whole is well."
—Plato

I have long held the belief that beyond our bodies and our emotions, there is also something else, something greater, at play. There is something working within each person's body that is intricately connected to the big picture and the world around us.

WE'LL SEE ...

There is a great Taoist story of an old farmer whose horse ran away. His neighbors came to him and said sympathetically "Such bad luck!" The farmer said simply, "We'll see."

A few days later, the horse came back, and brought with it three wild horses. The neighbors came again, telling him "How wonderful!" to which the old farmer answered, "We'll see."

Later that week his son, while trying to ride one of the wild horses, was thrown from it and broke his arm. The neighbors came to offer their sympathy, and the farmer shrugged and stated, "We'll see." The following day, military officers came to the village to draft young men for the army. Because his son had a broken arm, he did not have to join them.

The neighbors came again to offer their congratulations. "We'll see," said the farmer ...

7th Key: Trusting the Process

TAOISM—A BIG PICTURE PERSPECTIVE

Taoism is all about the big picture. Like the farmer in the story, Taoism is about trusting what comes, and being in the flow of life—allowing the ups and downs to happen without drama or force. Roughly translated, the *Tao Te Ching*, which is an ancient text that Taoism is based upon, means *the power of the yielding way*. In Taoism, you live in harmony—with the universe, with each other, and with your own body. There is groundedness in this way of living—a peace.

Chinese medicine is founded upon the spiritual philosophy of Taoism. They both embody the belief that everything is connected, and that there is a balance between opposing forces in the universe: *the cosmic dance of Yin and Yang*. Chinese medicine works to balance the energy of your body—without force—in order to support its harmonious and natural flow.

This holistic philosophy helps us see how our body relates to our lives. When we are sick, we tend to think that our body is getting in the way of what we are *supposed* to be doing. The truth is, everything is related. Our emotions and spiritual well-being fundamentally affect our body—and today's science is catching up to these ancient principles.

No matter what is happening in your life, you are always connected to the world around you. Your experiences are important. Your body holds *everything* in your life. What will help your body and spirit feel more connected, supported, alive, and free? What are the messages that are being conveyed through your body?

CAROL

My patient Carol luckily discovered a lump in her breast early. After her surgery she decided that life was giving her a message, and she delved into finding what it was. It made her review her life, specifically her marriage and her work.

Carol realized that she had been holding onto resentment and fear in her marriage. As she looked more deeply, she realized that she deeply loved her husband and he was perfect for her. By sharing her feelings and her fears with him, she gained the intimacy that she had been longing for, and they became closer than ever.

As a business owner, Carol had been a workaholic before her cancer. She changed her work hours so she could relax more, take care of herself, and spend more time with the people that she loved.

Carol shared her experiences through her writing. Her amazing sense of humor and playfulness helped her confront the places that weren't working in her marriage, life, and work and find what she needed to change. She even formed a cancer support group to help other women explore their healing process.

DEVELOP A WIDE LENS

When we separate and isolate the different aspects of our lives, we may overlook what is truly causing an issue. By pulling back and looking at the big picture, Chinese medicine is able to address disharmonies in our overall energy and create healing. That's why it can help us feel better even when we don't know what's going on.

Often, the idea of connecting the spirit and the body becomes distorted. People see sickness as a spiritual punishment or retributive karma, or a sign that God is angry or has abandoned them. These ideas are all based upon an assumption that when something "bad" happens to us, it means that somehow we've been bad, and that God or Life is vindictive.

Chinese medicine is much more forgiving in its perspective. It recognizes that certain external factors are beyond our control, and takes into account that we may not always be able to rule our emotional reactions. Acupuncture and other modalities help correct and align our energy, despite what may have happened to bring it out of balance in the first place. So, it takes into account our humanness and helps to reduce traumas that could cause further issues in the future.

You don't have to be Taoist to appreciate the magic and flow of life. And you don't have to receive acupuncture to experience the delicate balance inside of you and in the world around you. Part of the work of the 7th Key is to develop your wide-lens perspective, to learn to pull back and look at the different facets of your life, and how you are connected to the world around you.

Are there places that are obviously out of balance? Where do you need support? Beyond your body, what parts of you are crying out for healing? Is there a way for you to turn your gaze toward that which is beneficial, growing, and alive inside of you—rather than focusing so intently on the pain, the fear, and the disappointment? Imagine the difference you would feel in your body if someone was supporting you, taking care of you, and helping you every step of your day? Then, become that person.

> *"A human being is part of the whole, called by us as the Universe, a part limited in time and space. He experiences himself, his thoughts and feelings, as something separate from the rest—a kind of optical delusion of his consciousness."*
> —A<small>LBERT</small> E<small>INSTEIN</small>

Actions for the 4th Fundamental
Seeing the Big Picture

N<small>OTICE</small> B<small>EAUTY</small>
Pay attention to beauty. Whether flowers, music, food, or another person, notice the beauty in your life. This practice also naturally builds gratitude.

1. **Connect to Your Spirit**

    Whatever works for you, whatever you find that supports you—it is important that you make a practice of connecting to your spirit. Dedicate yourself to it. Keep it in your awareness. Maintaining the connection between your body and spirit and the world around you will help anchor you when times are tough.

    Here are some ways you can do this:
    - Some find that meditation and prayer offer the greatest solace and peace of mind to their spirit.
    - Being in nature.
    - Doing yoga or exercising can create a union between the body and spirit.
    - Intimacy, support groups, and sharing your feelings and thoughts with friends can be wonderfully balancing and cathartic.
    - And then there are creative endeavors; whether you are an artist or not, you can create something through words, or colors, or sounds, or even food, that helps express what you are experiencing.

2. **Wash a Dish Slowly**

    Take one dish that needs washing and hand wash it with a sponge. Cover every millimeter of the dish, and pay attention to each detail as you wash it. When you begin to rinse it, let the water run all over the dish, and make sure that each part is *completely* clear of soap, and that all soap is off your hands. With this method, it can take up to five minutes to wash a bowl! It teaches us to slow down, to be in the moment, and to vividly pay attention.

Conclusion

> *"This place where you are right now*
> *God circled on a map for you."*
> —Hafiz

What's Next?

In October, 2017, my community burned down. In the middle of the night, devastating wildfires raged through the hills and neighborhoods of Santa Rosa, CA. Thousands of people were awakened, with no warning, to escape from their homes just in time. Most of them left with nothing but the clothes on their back. More than 5,000 homes were burned to the ground, leaving so many in the community homeless and lost. The experience was devastating to everyone.

Loss, by its nature, is devastating. To lose everything, especially after you've worked so hard to build it, is heart-wrenching. To lose your faith in your ability to heal is also one of the worst possible experiences. If you've reached this point in the book, and you still don't feel that you are healed—the most important thing to remember is: *Keep going. There is hope.*

Even though my office building did not burn in the fires, it was in the middle of the evacuation zone, so I had to find other spaces to be able to keep helping my patients. At that time, it was vitally important to be able to provide a place for people to receive care and healing. Many in our community came together to offer services and be available to those whose homes were lost or had to be evacuated. As I am writing this, almost one year later, people are still in shock. It may take years to recover, but no matter the circumstances, I know that healing—from trauma, or loss, or illness, or fire—is a heroic journey.

For me, at that time, everything changed. In order to keep going and stay hopeful, I had to act, which is what I do when I feel powerless. I saw the trauma my patients and my community were going through, and I wanted to help more. I created an online event, The Disaster Recovery Summit, which is free to anyone whenever they need it (www.disasterrecoverysummit.com). It provides information from experts to help with the various emotional and physical aspects of recovering from a disaster of any sort. This provided an outlet for me to channel my pain and concerns about my patients, friends and community.

Through all that I've seen and experienced and discovered, I still believe in the power of hope—to keep going, no matter what. There is always more healing, more love, and more growth that can be done. No matter what has happened up to this point, hold onto the hope that you will find the person, the place, the treatment, or the idea that will help you heal. Don't give up on yourself. Whatever your journey looks like—it is heroic. Your path is important, and it has meaning, exactly as it is happening right now.

Conclusion

THE RETURN TO THE WORLD

"Energy and persistence conquer all things."
—BENJAMIN FRANKLIN

The final step of Campbell's Hero's Journey is the "Return to the World". This is when you go back to your "normal life" with the healing and mastery that you've gained, and find a way to thrive within the "ordinary" world. It means taking the wisdom and strength that you've acquired, and integrating it into your everyday life.

As Campbell states: *"Mastery leads to freedom from the fear of death, which in turn is the freedom to live."* Mastery does not mean perfection; it means that you have gained the skills to be able to understand, integrate, reflect upon, channel, and activate your energy. Mastery on the healing path means you don't give up. Health or healing is never a static state—it is flexible, dynamic, and moving—like Yin and Yang. Mastery is what you gain by willingly and bravely traveling on your healing journey.

Inside yourself, you are a different person than when you started this journey. You have faced your foes. You have become the hero of your own life. Your mission, as you return to the world, is to be true to that.

This final step can be the most difficult of all. It can take time to process your experiences sufficiently so that you can separate the wisdom gained from the ordeals endured. There is no preset timeline for this: it takes as long as it takes, and that is just the right amount of time.

HONOR YOUR JOURNEY

The point of going through your healing journey is to transform. In some ways, everything may look the same as it did before, but you know that you have changed. You understand your body better now. You can see the connections between your thoughts, emotions, and health. Your body will keep speaking to you and you'll keep on learning more and more all the time, because your body is now your guide.

The healing opportunity at this point, is to continue growing. Ask yourself, "What am I going to do now? Who was I before? Where was I happy? What new opportunities do I have?"

In life, we don't always get to feel like we've arrived, but in finishing this book, you've gone through a life-changing experience. Now, it's time to celebrate!

Create a ritual or a symbol of your healing. Do something special to honor the work that you've done and bring yourself solidly into the new. Build an altar, write a song, have a party, go to the ocean and say a prayer. Mark your arrival in this new place. It's an important step in moving forward.

How do you want to honor your journey?

Congratulations!
You are a miracle!!!

Appendix A

Chinese Medicine 101: An Introduction

UNDERSTANDING ENERGY: QI & CHINESE MEDICINE

In our day to day lives, we mostly think of energy in regard to transferral of energy. Sometimes we have a lot of energy, sometimes we're tired and need to restore it. Certain foods give us energy, while other foods deplete us. Sleep restores our energy, lack of sleep makes us cranky and tired. A fight with a loved one drains our energy, while a loving interaction makes us feel more vital, more alive.

Chinese medicine describes energy with a wider perspective. It asserts that our bodies are made up of energy, and that we are essentially energetic beings. The energy that gives us life is described as Qi (pronounced *chee*). Qi literally means breath—the air that is present in all living things—our life force, our vitality. It is what makes us who we are. *Qi* exists in rocks, rivers, bodies, light, computers—even thoughts, and emotions have Qi. It is universal, flowing through all things, and in a constant state of flux. Learning how Qi works, moves, and affects us is the basis of Chinese medicine.

Thousands of years ago, Chinese medicine practitioners discovered natural patterns of Qi that travel through the body in channels or pathways called

meridians. They identified 12 meridians that transport Qi everywhere in the body. It works like an energy distribution system. Each meridian is associated with a specific organ. Balanced Qi is essential to good health, so the work of Chinese medicine is to create and maintain balanced Qi in the body. Harmony in the body sustains health on every level; when your energy is balanced and flowing, you feel good—you are healthy, not only physically, but also emotionally and spiritually. Illness is the product of blocked, disrupted, or unbalanced Qi within the meridians.

According to Chinese medicine, everyone is born with a certain amount of Qi, which we inherit from our parents at the moment of conception! We can also acquire Qi based upon how we live our lives. There are countless things in life that affect the flow of Qi. From our thoughts and emotions, to the way we sit at work, to how we eat and exercise, to our daily interactions—everything that requires energy, (ie. everything!) can affect the balance of Qi in our bodies. Chinese Medicine practitioners work to regulate the circulation of Qi in the body through acupuncture, herbs, nutrition, and other modalities, adjusting the way that the energy moves, relieving imbalances, and impacting your health and life immeasurably.

Imagine that your body is an orchestra. When your body is functioning properly, it creates beautiful music and makes you feel good. Each "instrument" is vital to the symphony and affects the overall harmony of the music. If the clarinet is squeaking, the whole orchestra is affected. Similarly, if one thing is out of balance in your body, your entire body is affected. You cannot separate a symptom from the other parts of your body.

In an orchestra, if the squeaky clarinet is removed, there has to be a shift in the composition of the music in order to create the same sense of sound. If the composer and the orchestra are focused only on fixing the squeaky clarinet, the music will suffer. The problem needs to be addressed, but not at the cost of the whole. Your body, like an orchestra, works in concert, so that each part—your brain, your organs, the fuel you take in, your daily experi-

Appendix A—Chinese Medicine 101: An Introduction

ences—*everything* affects how the music sounds, and how you feel at the end of the day.

ACUPUNCTURE

The physical practice of acupuncture involves inserting thin needles into certain points on the body in order to change energy movement. When the flow of energy in the body is balanced, cells restore themselves to their natural state, and the body can heal itself naturally. There are more than 300 acupuncture points on the body and each one has a different effect.

Most needles used in conventional medicine are beveled - so they cut the tissues as they go through, which is why they hurt. Acupuncture needles don't hurt because they are designed more like pins to move through the tissues without cutting them (and of course, they're much thinner than pins!). In the US, the FDA approved acupuncture needles as a medical device in 1996. Prior to that, they were considered an "experimental medical device" and a great deal of research was done before it was approved.

Studies show that when acupuncture is used for pain, endorphins are released, allowing the body to feel less pain. For infertility, acupuncture helps the body produce more hormones. For bronchitis or flu symptoms it has been found to increase the immune cells needed to fight the virus. In studies of people with ulcers, it helps the stomach balance acid production. One of the most important things that acupuncture does, is to help reduce stress, which by itself is a major cause of most illness.

In 1979 there was a World Health Organization inter-regional conference in Beijing determine the efficacy of acupuncture. And in 1997 the NIH—National Institute of Health approved acupuncture as a viable treatment option for various health conditions. It was approved as a technique for many conditions including: pain of all sorts, headaches, TMJ, strokes, menstrual problems, fertility problems, respiratory infections such as sore throats, bronchitis and asthma, sleep disorders, and digestive problems including ulcers, gastritis, colitis, constipation and irritable bowel syndrome.

When I made my first acupuncture appointment, I had nothing to treat. I was not in pain or sick, but I felt that it was time for me to experience the medicine that had already changed my life.

By some miraculous twist of fate, the day that I walked in for my first acupuncture session I had a terrible migraine. I felt so sick! I'd had migraines in the past, so I knew what they felt like. For me, they usually took three days to go away regardless of what I did.

My acupuncturist put in the needles. I was lying on my stomach and there were needles in my neck, my back, my arms and my legs. At one point, I was looking down at my arm, and one of the needles began moving all on its own! The needle was on the back of my forearm pointing towards my head, and as I watched, it rotated towards my fingers. I wasn't moving my body, and no one was touching me. I didn't understand what was happening but I felt that it had something to do with energy moving in my body.

A few hours after the treatment, my headache was completely gone! This affirmed not only my belief in Chinese medicine, but my faith in miracles! I had just had an experience that felt miraculous to me.

After that, I had many more acupuncture treatments. Each one showed me more deeply the incredible healing that it provides. One time, I had a severe flu. I was so sick that I tried to cancel my appointment for acupuncture. I had a terrible sore throat, high fever, and aches. My practitioner told me to come in anyway, and within two hours of my treatment, my sore throat and fever were gone!

Chinese medicine is the best system I have found for explaining energy as it applies to the body. I was a believer before I had even experienced it, but the practice of acupuncture and Chinese medicine proved to be even more incredible than I had thought.

Appendix A—Chinese Medicine 101: An Introduction

BEYOND ANATOMY

FRANK

Frank came in to see me with lower back pain. He was a business owner and under a great deal of stress when I first met him. Professionally, everything in his life was in upheaval. He did not have the employees or the support that he needed, and he had to move out of his current office and had not yet found a new location. Overall, he felt his business was struggling. He was completely overwhelmed—and with overwhelm came fear, the most common stressor for most of us.

Through acupuncture and herbs, I worked on Frank's kidneys and on his stress. Within one month, everything in his professional life had turned around. He had found an office, had hired staff that he needed, and his business was again accelerating.

Chinese medicine asserts that if we become more balanced in our bodies, there will be a greater flow to all of our experiences. By balancing Frank's kidney energy through acupuncture his whole life was affected. After just four sessions, he was able to feel more balanced so that his life could flow more easily.

Much of Western scientific research asserts that acupuncture works simply because the points are near anatomic structures that respond to the stimulus of the needles. Research focuses upon anatomy, because it is can be empirically proven. The meridians follow blood vessels and nerves and lymphatic channels, therefore, acupuncture is simply stimulating the flow in those pathways. While this is definitely true, there is so much more to Chinese medicine than simple anatomy. Some of the effects of acupuncture treatments are beyond the physical, and these effects can be more difficult to scientifically quantify.

The spiritual and emotional effects of acupuncture are not strictly due to anatomy. Over the years, I've worked with people who have come in during a difficult time in their lives, and they don't just get better physically, they experience a reorganization of their lives that helps them feel better on every level. When someone is experiencing deep grief, acupuncture can calm the emotions. When I do a PTSD (Post Traumatic Stress Disorder) treatment, it can help my client overcome the trauma, sometimes as though it never happened. Not everyone attributes the changes that they experience in their lives to acupuncture, but I've worked with hundreds of people who have had dramatic shifts in their lives after they came to my office. These shifts are not merely physical.

Diagnosis

Chinese medicine practitioners use several methods to guide their understanding of the body. In addition to an in depth history and inquiry, there are two methods of diagnosis that are specifically unique to Chinese medicine: measuring the pulse of the patient, and discerning the appearance of the tongue. Together, these methods allow practitioners to assess which imbalance is playing a part in your physical symptoms.

By feeling the pulse, we can tell what is going on with 12 different internal organs. As you might imagine, it takes a lot of practice to be good at it. We feel the pulse in 3 positions on each wrist. Each position represents a different organ system. What is important is not how fast the pulse is, but how it feels. For example, a pulse can be scattered, hollow, faint, or long, and all of these will help me understand which organs have imbalance.

The appearance of the tongue also helps with diagnosis. A healthy tongue is a robust pink with a thin white coat and no extra markings. The front represents the heart and lungs. The middle represents the stomach and spleen, the back the kidneys, and the sides represent the liver/gallbladder. If the tongue is bright red, or yellow, or if it has spots or a thick coating, these are all indications of an imbalance.

In Chinese medicine, physical issues are diagnosed based upon the patterns of energy or disharmony in the body. It is based on the movement of

Appendix A—Chinese Medicine 101: An Introduction

opposites. 5,000 years ago, when Chinese medicine was first initiated, they did not have microscopes or chemistry labs. Disease was described by how the body behaves, and it was viewed in ways that are similar to how we witness the weather. Certain diseases were described as cold, damp, hot, windy or dry. There are eight fundamental patterns of energy imbalance: heat & cold, internal & external, deficiency & excess, and yin & yang.

ELEMENTS, ORGANS, AND SEASONS

As I have previously described in this book, each organ has a pathway of energy, or *a meridian,* that travels throughout your body, and there are many different functions attributed to each organ than what we commonly understand in Western medicine. In addition, they also have many other characteristics and qualities. Each organ has a time of year, a time of day, an element, a color, a sense organ, a flavor, a body tissue, and emotional and spiritual functions. By knowing these things, you can tell when you're out of balance, and which organ might be affected. Everything is about balance and creating harmony in your body, and energy patterns. Even your cravings can tell you more about your organs and where you might be suffering an imbalance. When you live according to the principles of Chinese medicine, you find yourself feeling more in harmony with your life and yourself.

I have included a chart (on the next page) that shows which organ goes with which time of year, element, color, etc, so that you can see how they flow.

YIN ORGAN	KIDNEY	LIVER	HEART	SPLEEN	LUNG
ELEMENT	Water	Wood	Fire	Earth	Metal
EMOTION	Fear	Anger	Joy	Worry/ Anxiety	Sadness/ Grief
YANG ORGAN	Bladder	Gall Bladder	Small Intestines	Stomach	Large Intestines
SEASON	Winter	Spring	Summer	Late Summer	Fall
CLIMATIC QI	Cold	Wind	Heat	Damp	Dryness
SENSE ORGAN	Ears	Eyes	Tongue	Mouth	Nose
BODY TISSUE	Bone	Sinews	Blood Vessels	Muscles	Skin
COLOR	Black	Green	Red	Yellow	White
TASTE	Salty	Sour	Bitter	Sweet	Spicy

Organ Clock and Seasons

All organs have a time of day and a time of year when they are more prevalent. Paying attention to the cycles of time with each organ can optimize your healing process. For example, fall is the time of year for the lungs, and they regulate the immune system, if you have an immune imbalance, fall is a very important time to be getting lots of rest, eating well, and taking immune supporting supplements.

Organ Clock

3 am–5 am

Lung: You may find that you wake up during these times if you are struggling with grief or sorrow. It is also a good time to get up and meditate and breathe deeply.

Appendix A—Chinese Medicine 101: An Introduction

5 am–7 am

    Large Intestine: If you have weak overall energy—your large intestines will also be weak and you might have diarrhea or intestinal cramping at this time of day.

7 am–9 am

    Stomach: This is the best time to eat a healthy and hearty break- fast.

9 am–11 am

    Spleen: If your digestion is good, you might be able to concentrate best at this time of day—because the spleen regulates your ability to concentrate.

11 am–1 pm

    Heart: The heart and small intestine are organs that work together. It's a good time of day to get together with friends—the heart deals with connection. If you have heart issues you might notice them especially at this time of day.

1 pm–3 pm

    Small Intestine: The small intestine separates the clear from the turbid, it's job in digestion, so if you are digesting your food at this time, that's a good thing. It is also a time of day that you can organize thoughts and get mental work done, (sorting the clear from the turbid mentally as well.)

3 pm–5 pm

Urinary Bladder: The bladder is paired with the kidneys, so you might notice a dip in energy during the 3-7 pm time frame if you are deficient in kidney energy. It is also a time of day for taking a rest/nap for restoring your energy. If you are kidney deficient you will feel more tired now.

5 pm–7 pm

Kidneys: If you have low kidney energy you will be more tired at this time of day. This also reflects low adrenal hormones.

7 pm–9 pm

Pericardium: To support the pericardium, this is the time to do something gentle to help you ease into sleep, such as meditation, light stretching, reading, or cuddling.

9 pm–11 pm

Triple Burner: Metabolism and blood vessels are most prevalent during this time, it would not be a good time to eat a meal—but it would be a great time to be digesting one. We should think about going to sleep during this time—having an earlier bed time in the winter, and staying up a little later in summer.

11 pm–1 am

Gall Bladder: This is a great time to go to bed and begin sleeping. The gallbladder rules decision making so if you are trying to make a decision, going to sleep now is going to help regenerate. It also rules the ligaments and tendons, so resting now can help them heal.

1 am–3 am

Liver: Time of detoxing—sleeping during this time is great for regenerating and clearing liver energy. You may find that you wake up during this time if you have repressed anger or long-standing resentment.

Seasons

Fall

Lungs/large Intestine: As I've already mentioned—this is a great time to boost your immune system and to do a cleanse to get ready for winter.

Winter

Kidneys/Urinary Bladder: This is the time of year that you will feel the lowest in energy. I usually don't recommend cleansing at this time of year (which is when many people want to cleanse for the new year). This is the time of year I recommend resting and hibernating-not over doing it.

Spring

Liver/Gallbladder: This is when the sap starts flowing and energy increases. It's the best time of year for a cleanse. Since the liver regulates the emotion of anger, you might notice that you're more irritable at this time of year if your liver is out of balance.

Early Summer

Heart/Small Intestine: This is when summer heat begins. This is a good time of year to get lots of cardiovascular exercise because fire rules the heart, and the heat of summer can fuel the fire.

Late Summer, Harvest
Spleen/Stomach: This is the time of connection to the earth and there is nothing better than harvest to experience that. It's a good time to pay attention to how your digestion is working. If you have trouble it's especially important to eat slowly, and chew food well. This is also a good time to work with blood sugar issues if you have them.

TWO ADDITIONAL ORGANS

There are two additional organs in Chinese medicine I have not yet discussed in detail: the pericardium and the triple burner. While the pericardium is known in Western science—it is the double layered sac of connective tissue that surrounds the heart (the heart envelope)—the triple burner is not recognized, partly because it is not a physical organ. Interestingly, just in the last year (2017) an article came out talking about a "new" organ system that had been discovered, which fits the description of the triple burner. Following is a description of each.

TRIPLE BURNER

This organ-energy system, is called the 'Minister of Dykes and Dredges' and is responsible for the movement and transformation of various solids and fluids throughout the body, as well as for the production and circulation of nourishing energy (*ying chee*) and protective energy (*wei chee*). It is not a single self-contained organ, but rather a functional energy system involved in regulating the activities of other organs. It is composed of three parts, known as 'burners', each connected with one of the body's three main cavities: chest, abdomen, and pelvis. An ancient Chinese medical text states: 'The Upper Burner controls intake, the Middle Burner controls transformation, the Lower Burner controls elimination.'

The Upper Burner runs from the base of the tongue to the entrance to the stomach and controls the intake of air, food, and fluids. It harmonizes the functions of heart and lungs, governs respiration, and regulates the distribution of protective energy to the body's external surfaces.

The Middle Burner runs from the entrance to the stomach down to its exit at the pyloric valve (the junction between the stomach and the small intestines) and controls digestion by harmonizing the functions of stomach, spleen, and pancreas. It is responsible for extracting nourishing energy from food and fluids and distributing it via the meridian system to the lungs and other parts of the body.

The Lower Burner runs from the pyloric valve down to the anus and urinary tract and is responsible for separating the pure from the impure products of digestion, absorbing nutrients, and eliminating solid and liquid wastes. It harmonizes the functions of liver, kidney, bladder, and large and small intestines and also regulates sexual and reproductive functions.

Some medical researchers believe that the Triple Burner is associated with the hypothalamus, the part of the brain, which regulates appetite, digestion, fluid balance, body temperature, heartbeat, blood pressure, and other basic autonomous functions.

Emotionally the triple burners help regulate the consciousness and move the emotional energy of other organs. For example, liver stagnation can cause depression, the triple warmer helps balance it.

PERICARDIUM

In Chinese medicine—the pericardium is responsible for protecting the heart. The heart is the emperor of all the organs and needs protection. Many of the physical functions we attribute to our hearts in the west, are attributed to the pericardium in Chinese medicine. So, when someone has a heart attack, or congestive heart failure, or an arrhythmia—these are functions of the pericardium.

Within us, if the heart is not well protected, love and joy disappear; sadness and fear arise. We experience internal disorder and can neither love ourselves nor be open to the love of others. We feel vulnerable, easily hurt, and "heartbroken." We lose our feeling of connection to life and to others, which pervades everything. In the other extreme, we may shut down and overprotect ourselves. Instead of appropriate opening, the fear of being hurt shuts everyone out, making us feel separate and isolated. When the Pericardium is doing its job, it keeps out those who would do harm and allows entry to those who are trustworthy, loving, fun, and good for our energy.

Importantly—points on the pericardium meridian are often used to help treat people when they have issues with relationships with other people. They are also used to treat the physical symptoms of heart issues.

Appendix B

Lifestyle Suggestions

LIST OF BASIC SUPPLEMENTS

Every individual is different and therefore will most likely require different supplements, but there are a few basic nutrients that lay the foundation for good health.

Some people might disagree as to the need for multivitamins, but in my experience, most people don't get enough adequate nutrients in their diet to support their bodies well. Add to that, if you have a stressful job, commute to work, overdo exercise, don't get outside enough, and other things, you will need some support of your body.

Please see my free pdf booklet on how to choose supplements—*hearttoheartmedicalcenter.com*—for extensive information about ingredients and quality of ingredients you should choose.

Here Is a List of the Basics That I Think Most People Should Have

*A good **Multi-vitamin** should contain the following:*

a. Folate: 400-800 mcg
b. Thiamine: 25-50 mg
c. Riboflavin: 25-50 mg
d. Niacin: 100 mg
e. Vitamin B6: 25-50 mg
f. B12: 100-500 mcg
g. Biotin: 200-800 mcg
h. Pantothenic Acid: 100 mg
i. Zinc: 15 mg
j. Selenium: 100-200 mcg
k. Chromium: 100-200 mcg
l. Manganese: 5 mg
m. Molybdenum: 50 mcg
n. Iodine: 100 mcg
o. Vitamin A: 5000-10000 IU
p. Vitamin C: 150-1000 mg
q. Vitamin D: 1000-5000 IU
r. Vitamin E: 100-400 IU
s. Vitamin K: 100-250 mcg
t. Copper: 1 mg (this might be contra-indicated for someone with copper excess or cancer)
u. Calcium: It's a large molecule and might not fit into a one-a-day multiple vitamin
v. Magnesium: It's a large molecule and the amount needed varies. I recommend this as a separate supplement.

Appendix B—Lifestyle Suggestions

1. **Magnesium:** This is required for more than 400 chemical reactions in the body. Most people are magnesium deficient. I recommend that everyone take at least 400 mg a day. Some may need more.

2. **Omega 3 Fatty Acids:** Omega 3 fatty acids have many benefits including helping balance the triangle of wellness—the immune system, hormones, and nervous system. They provide a long list of other benefits including preventing dry eyes, decreasing symptoms of arthritis, heart protection, and helping with the symptoms of ADHD. They are essential to wellness on every level. The minimum amount should be 500 mg of a combination of EPA and DHA, but various health conditions require more. Omega 3 fatty acids are available in some foods, most especially fatty fish, walnuts, flax seeds, chia seeds, organic eggs, meats that were raised in their natural environment (i.e. grass fed and finished beef, wild game, etc.), and algae. Omega 3 from vegetarian sources except for algae do not contain DHA, which is the omega 3 that affects the nervous system. I recommend omega 3 supplements because it's hard to make sure you get enough of them in your diet, and they are so essential.

3. **Vitamin D:** Vitamin D is so important that we now measure levels in our blood to make sure there is enough. It is needed for the immune system, hormones, and nervous system. Many people say it's hard to get enough from sun exposure alone, but I think that's because most people don't get enough sun exposure on a daily basis. It also gets used up faster when you're under stress. Depending on your blood level, your requirement will vary. Most people need from 2000-5000 IU a day.

4. **Probiotics:** This is an area of controversy in my mind. Many people do OK with probiotics and have no side effects from them. But if you have chronic digestive problems, you may not do well with probiotics because

your microbiome might not work right. So we can't say that EVERYONE needs probiotics, because at least half the people I see have issues with their digestion.

LIST OF EMERGENCY SYMPTOMS

Below is a list of symptoms that should prompt you to consider going to the emergency room, or at least calling your doctor or the local ER advice nurse to figure out if you need to go. Keep in mind, we have no way of knowing for sure when you are in a life-or-death situation, but the following are symptoms that may indicate a severe problem that will need immediate attention.

1. Shortness of breath.
2. Sudden onset chest pain or upper abdominal pain that lasts more than two minutes. It can be sharp, dull, radiating, or going down your arm. If a sudden chest pain lasts, please call 911 or an ambulance for immediate assistance.
3. Any sudden or severe pain.
4. Sudden fainting/or passing out for no apparent reason.
5. Severe abdominal pain that increases with breathing, movement, or light touch. This can be pain that lasts any length of time, but is marked by not getting better over the course of a few minutes to an hour.
6. Uncontrollable bleeding—including menstrual bleeding.
7. An accident that results in you not being able to move some part of your body or having severe pain any place that you can't explain. Remember, an accident may raise your adrenaline levels and cause you to not really know what your abilities are. Let someone call an ambulance if there is ANY question.
8. Sudden onset of one-sided weakness anywhere in your body.
9. Blood pressure that is too high. Higher than 160/120 would be an emergency.

Appendix B—Lifestyle Suggestions

10. Feeling suicidal.
11. Racing heart rate that occurs suddenly and unexpectedly and doesn't go away with a few deep breaths. If your pulse is more than 120 beats per minute at rest, you should call for help.
12. Coughing or vomiting blood.
13. Severe or persistent vomiting or diarrhea.
14. Unusual abdominal pain.
15. Unexplained seizures.
16. The worst headache of your life, especially if it's sudden.

LIST OF TESTS THAT SHOULD BE DONE

As always, I recommend labs based on what I need to know about a person's health, but there are some labs that are helpful for many conditions. I will include here labs that I often order when I see a new patient, and why.

THE BASICS

There are some basic labs that most doctors would order, and which are usually covered by insurance depending on what insurance you have.

These include:
CBC: Complete blood count.
Lipid Panel: It measures cholesterol and the components associated with cholesterol.
Chem 14: A panel of basic chemistry of your body that includes liver tests, kidney tests, electrolytes, and blood sugar.
Hemoglobin A1C, or Glycohemoglobin: It measures the average blood sugar in red blood cells over the past 12 weeks or so. When elevated, it can mean that you have a higher blood sugar than normal.
TSH, Free T3, Free T4, TPO Antibodies: It is some basic thyroid labs that can indicate what is happening to your thyroid.

Insulin: Can show if you are insulin resistant.

GGT: This test shows the level of toxicity in your body.

Iron, Ferritin, TIBC: This test shows the status of iron in your body.

HORMONE TESTING: DUTCH TEST

This is a dried urine test performed four times in the course of a day by peeing on a filter paper and letting it dry, which can show how your adrenal hormones are doing. There are more than 20 adrenal hormones.

There are several unique things about this test. It shows not only the levels of various adrenal hormones, it also shows how your body uses those hormones, which can be helpful in figuring out treatment options. It shows how the body detoxifies hormones as well. And there are several additional bonuses, which include looking at B12, B6 and some neurotransmitters, so it represents the state of your adrenals well. One surprising thing in comparison to previously popular saliva testing for hormones is that we now know you may have a low cortisol but could still have a high metabolized cortisol. It is changing the definition of adrenal fatigue.

STOOL TEST

These tests are used to look at your digestion and see if you have various issues. It can show infections, the state of your microbiome, whether you digest your food or not, and the level of inflammation in your gut. I've done these tests for more than 20 years on my patients, and my current favorite test is called GI MAP test, which looks at the DNA of various infectious agents and can show me what is going on in your guts at a deeper level. Over the years, I've found that many stool tests don't show the infections a person has, even when it's pretty clear there is some sort of infection based on their symptoms. This test has been the best at finding them, of all the tests I've performed.

Appendix B—Lifestyle Suggestions

NUTRIEVAL: GENOVA LABS

This test is a urine and blood test that shows the nutritional state of your body, including B vitamins, amino acids, fatty acids, minerals, how your cells produce energy, if there are digestive problems, toxins and your ability to detoxify, and heavy metals. It's a very thorough test which can help reveal a root cause of your health concerns while also allowing me to help you get your nutritional state more balanced.

DIETARY SUGGESTIONS

Diet varies for every person and every health condition, so these recommendations are very generic. As I've mentioned before, there are millions of diet books, and many people have followed many different diets. Here are suggestions that I make to almost everyone I see.

The primary focus of a healthy diet is *always* to eat as many vegetables as possible. Wherever you go, whatever you eat, look for creative ways to get more veggies. When I have a hamburger, I order broccoli as a side dish instead of fries. When you go to a restaurant, try to order a dish that has lots of vegetables. When you make food at home, you can chop up a variety of vegetables and quickly steam or roast them. Dr. Terry Wahl, who healed herself of MS and then proceeded to do a study showing the benefits of eating vegetables, suggests 9 cups of vegetables a day for healing. I suggest that you try to make vegetables more than 50% of your diet—and if you are ill, they should be even more, up to 80%. One great way to incorporate vegetables into your diet is to have a *Vitamixer*, and blend a variety of them into a drink every day.

The next ingredient of a healthy diet is protein, preferably at every meal. Protein helps you stay grounded and keeps your blood sugar stable. It supplies nutrition for your brain and hormone systems. Depending on your body type or food preferences, protein can be derived from many sources. Some people focus primarily on meat for their protein, while vegans and vegetarians use combinations of grains, legumes, beans, nuts, and vegetables for their protein.

Good fats should be the next focus on your diet, and are necessary for the neurotransmitters and hormones that keep things functioning. Deficiency of good oils is connected to high cholesterol, ADD, ADHD, PMS, fatigue, and menopausal symptoms, as well as depression and other psychological problems. Try to include good fats in every meal. Nuts, avocados, olive oil, nut oil, and coconut oil are sources of good fat. "Bad" fats, including partially hydrogenated vegetable oils (aka shortening or trans fats) are not nutritionally beneficial, actually can be harmful, and should be avoided when possible.

In general, I recommend you eat breakfast within one hour of getting up, especially if you have adrenal issues. When you have high cortisol levels, having a high-protein breakfast within one hour of getting up in the morning helps you stabilize your blood sugar, and helps control your cortisol levels. As much as people love to eat sweet things often, this is the worst thing to have in the morning.

Intermittent fasting: There is a lot of science about intermittent fasting for helping balance blood sugar, support weight loss, and heal digestive disorders. You can find a lot of information about this online, but I suggest that you work yourself toward eating your last meal between 6-7pm and then not eat anything else until the following morning. This alone will make a difference in your blood sugar and help your digestion.

EXERCISE

When you've been ill for a long time, exercise is probably the last thing on your mind. It may be difficult for you to just get out of bed in the morning. Eventually, movement and exercise will be a part of your healing process, and I like to think of it early in the process. Movement is so essential to healing our bodies. Even if you don't have the energy to get up out of bed, some gentle movements every day will help heal your body.

Appendix B—Lifestyle Suggestions

When you are involved in a healing process, it's best to figure out what type of movement or exercise to do with the help of a professional who knows the state of your health. You may just start with something like a short walk, 5 minutes a day. Or you may do some gentle stretches in your bed in the morning.

As with diets, there are so many ways to exercise. Every injury, and many chronic diseases, will improve with exercise. If you have a back injury, special exercises can strengthen the support structure of your spine, so you are less likely to reinjure it. Even if you've broken a bone, such as your wrist or ankle, exercise is what will help it heal in the long run. Initially you have to stop moving that fracture so it will set, but then you need to exercise it to heal it.

I have so many patients who have been injured in an accident and have not fully recovered. I continuously encourage them to get their body moving again. Many are afraid because of the pain they feel; they think the pain will increase with more movement. At first, the pain may indeed increase, but if you never start exercising again, you will never get better. With time, the pain will diminish. Post-injury exercise should be guided by someone who knows which movements will help heal and strengthen the body.

Fibromyalgia is a chronic pain condition that causes muscles to ache all over the body. It seems to be related to hormonal and sleep disorders. The right exercise is part of the long-term solution to the problem. Arthritis also improves with exercise.

For years, I believed that if a group of muscles was tight, you should not do anything to strengthen them because then they would only get tighter. I learned through personal experience that muscle tension is often due to weakness of the muscles in the back. Chronic shoulder and neck tension can occur when we do nothing to strengthen the back muscles that hold up our bodies. Weight training of the upper body and back is very helpful if you have problems in this area.

Walking is a great way to connect with nature while also moving your body. Studies show that we should walk a minimum of 5,000 steps a day. There is a form of yoga called restorative yoga where you lie on the floor supported by props in certain positions for up to 15 minutes per pose. It is extremely healing and relaxing, and can be done when you have extreme fatigue or weakness. It's also useful for calming severe anxiety. Other wonderful, gentle, whole-body exercises are Tai Chi, Pilates, or Qi Gong. Each of them can be modified to be very gentle for people who are struggling. Qi Gong is an ancient form of movement in Chinese tradition that is particularly used for healing. There are particular forms of movement that can heal each organ.

Appendix C
Resources

Bannerman, R., MD. (July-Sept. 1980). The World Health Organization Viewpoint On Acupuncture. *American Journal of Acupuncture, 8*(3).

Cigna Corporation. (2018, May 1). *New Cigna Study Reveals Loneliness at Epidemic Levels in America* [Press release]. Retrieved from www.cigna.com/newsroom/news-releases/2018/new-cigna-study-reveals-loneliness-at-epidemic-levels-in-america.

Collingwood, J. (2016, July 17). How Does Mood Affect Immunity? Retrieved from psychcentral.com/lib/how-does-mood-affect-immunity/.

Dahlke, Reudiger, MD. "Disease As the Language of the Soul." Retrieved from: www.dahlke.at.

Dhabhar, F. S., Malarkey, W. B., Neri, E., & Mcewen, B. S. (2012). Stress-induced redistribution of immune cells—From barracks to boulevards to battlefields: A tale of three hormones – Curt Richter Award Winner. *Psychoneuroendocrinology, 37*(9), 1345-1368. doi:10.1016/j.psyneuen.2012.05.008.

Explore (NY). 2008 Jul-Aug;4(4):235-43. doi: 10.1016/j.explore.2008.04.002. Compassionate intention as a therapeutic intervention by partners of cancer patients: effects of distant intention on the patients' autonomic nervous system.

Radin D1, Stone J, Levine E, Eskandarnejad S, Schlitz M, Kozak L, Mandel D, Hayssen G.

Felitti, V. J., Anda, R. F., Nordenberg, D., Williamson, D. F., Spitz, A. M., Edwards, V., . . . Marks, J. S. (1998). Relationship of Childhood Abuse and Household Dysfunction to Many of the Leading Causes of Death in Adults. *American Journal of Preventive Medicine, 14*(4), 245-258. doi:10.1016/s0749-3797(98)00017-8.

Fottrell, Q. (2018, August 18). Why loneliness can damage your health. Retrieved from www.marketwatch.com/story/america-has-a-big-loneliness-problem-2018-05-02.

Grimm, R., Jr., Spring, K., & Dietz, N. (2007). Study by the National Corporation for Community Service.

Hamilton, D. R., Ph.D. (2016, May 06). 6 Reasons Why The Love Hormone Is Good For You. Retrieved from www.huffingtonpost.com/david-r-hamilton-phd/6-reasons-why-the-love-ho_b_7171514.html.

HeartMath Institute. (n.d.). Research FAQs. Retrieved from www.heartmath.org/support/faqs/research/.

HeartMath Institute. (n.d.). Chapter 06: Energetic Communication. Retrieved from www.heartmath.org/research/science-of-the-heart/energetic-communication/.

Kiecolt-Glaser, J. K., Ph.D, Loving, T. J., Ph.D., Stowell, J. R., Ph.D., Malarkey, W. B., MD, Lemeshow, S., Ph.D., Dickenson, S. A., MAS, & Glaser, R., Ph.D. (2005). Hostile Marital Interactions, Proinflammatory Cytokine Production, and Wound Healing. *Archives of General Psychiatry, 62*(12). doi:10.1001/archpsyc.62.12.1377.

Marche, S. (2018, July 14). Is Facebook Making Us Lonely? Retrieved from www.theatlantic.com/magazine/archive/2012/05/is-facebook-making-us-lonely/308930/.

McCraty, R., Ph.D., Atkinson, M., & D. T., B.A. (2003). Modulation of DNA Conformation by Heart-Focused Intention. *HeartMath Research Center: Institute of HeartMath, 03*(008).

Mohd, R. S. (2008). Life Event, Stress and Illness. *Malaysian Journal of Medical Sciences, 15*(4), 9-18.

Rapp, S. (2016, March 09). Why Success Always Starts With Failure. Retrieved from 99u.com/articles/7072/why-success-always-starts-with-failure.

Rimer, S., & Drexler, M. (2014, February 19). Happiness & health. Retrieved from www.hsph.harvard.edu/news/magazine/happiness-stress-heart-disease/.

Saslow, R. (2011, February 07). Health benefits of falling and staying in love. Retrieved from www.washingtonpost.com/wp-dyn/content/article/2011/02/07/AR2011020703564.html.

Thaik, D. C. (2013, July 06). The Healing Powers Of Love. Retrieved from www.huffingtonpost.com/dr-cynthia-thaik/love-health-benefits_b_3131370.html.

Torpy, J. M., MD, C. L., MA, & Glass, R. M., MD. (2007). Chronic Stress and the Heart. *Journal of the American Medical Association, 298*(14). doi:10.1001/jama.298.14.1722.

Index

7 Keys

1st Key
Chapter 1, 61–94
cornerstone of the 7 Keys, 65–66
defining the 1st Key/healing energy of love, 62–63
fundamentals of 1st Key, 65–67
science of love, 64–65

2nd Key
Chapter 2, 95–127
defining the 2nd Key, 97–98
fundamentals of 2nd Key, 99–100
medicine, 121
surgery, 120
Triangle of Wellness, 99, 102

3rd Key
Chapter 3, 128–160
defining the 3rd Key, 128–129
elimination diet, 147–150
fundamentals of 3rd Key, 130–132

4th Key
Chapter 4, 161–191
defining the 4th Key, 164
fundamentals of the 4th Key, 164–165
in relation to symptoms, 164, 173, 179–188
listening despite fear, 188–189

5th Key
Chapter 5, 192–224
defining the 5th Key, 197, 207
fundamentals of the 5th Key, 164–165
heart–joy, 207–208
kidneys–fear, 212
liver–anger, 211–212
lungs–grief, 209–210
spleen–worry, 210–211
releasing emotions, exercises, 204–205, 222–223

6th Key
Chapter 6, 225–248
defining the 6th Key, Hero's journey, 227
fundamentals of the 6th Key,
Growth Mindset, 236–237
hope, 247
persistence–yang, 231, 232
patience–yin, 231, 233

7th Key
Chapter 7, 249–280
defining the 7th Key, 254, 255, 256

fundamentals of the 7th Key, 256–257
alchemical nature, 254–255, 256
checking the facts, 268–69
wide-lens perspective, 278–279

A

acupuncture
2nd Key, as part of, 97–98
description of, 287-288
emotions and energy, balancing, 37, 75, 176, 206, 278
history, study of, 32
needles, 287
NIH approval, 287–88
PTSD, treating, 79, 203–204, 226, 290
qi, aiding in circulation of, 40, 286
spiritual and emotional effects, 289–90
stuck energy, helping to release, 86, 222

adrenals
adrenal fatigue, 226
adrenal hormone testing, 108–9, 304
breakfast as stabilizing, 306
cortisol, produced by adrenal gland, 72–74
kidneys, ruling, 175, 187

Adverse Childhood Events (ACEs), 112, 201

Aikido, 88, 157–58

allergies
cautionary note, 151
dairy allergy, 162–63
gluten sensitivity, 145–46
hormones, allergies causing imbalance in,103
immune system health, 106
organs and related allergy symptoms, 186–87
PTSD causing allergies, 203
sleep apnea resulting from allergies, 121

anger (also see *liver*)
chronic stress manifesting as anger, 213
depression, underlying anger, 187
exercises to release anger, 204–205
gallbladder, ruling, 211, 217
immune system, anger depleting, 105
LIVER, ruling 36–37, 154, 183–184, 295
physical exercise, best way to release, 211, 221
physical symptoms of, 184, 202, 207, 211
in organ-pairings chart, 292
redirecting anger, 71, 100, 174, 204, 216, 218, 221, 255
releasing, support 154, 211–212, 234
sleep issues, 188
surrendering, 272

anxiety (also see *spleen, stomach*)
antibiotics use, contributing factor, 114
chronic inflammation, linked with, 73
chronic stress, manifesting as, 213
cortisol, affecting levels, 73, 138
differentiating anxiety from true alarm signals, 81
dysfunctions of the heart, causing, 208
exercises to shift anxiety, 82–84, 211
exercises to process, 204–205
in organ-pairings chart, 292
oxytocin, anxiety reduced by release of, 73
PTSD, as a symptom of, 203
spleen, 95–96, 176, 182, 210, 292

Index

stomach aches, related to, 139, 182
sudden anxiety, examining, 69
yoga poses for anxiety, 211, 308
worry, stomach connected to, 137, 171

B
blood pressure and hypertension
high blood pressure, 80, 89, 184, 202, 213, 302
lowering blood pressure, 73

bones
broken bones, 307
kidneys, ruling, 105, 175, 185, 212
in organ-pairings chart, 292

breakfast
protein, 138, 142, 306
timing, consistency, 108, 144, 147, 306

breath work
in Coherence practice, 77
deep breathing, exercises, 82, 84, 181, 209, 223, 292
fear response, effect on breathing, 80
in *Katsugen Undo* practice, 88–89
nervous system and, 108, 209
parasympathetic nervous system, resetting, 82
qi as breath, 39
seasonal breathing exercises, 144
breathing into tension, 173

Brown, Brené, 90

C
Campbell, Joseph, 47, 271, 283

cancer
2nd Key, 99
breast cancer, 68–69, 126, 220–21, 277–78
chronic inflammation, linked with, 73
copper supplements, 300
fear, courage/discernment, 79, 81, 189
gene testing and, 116–17
loneliness and, 89
love and the healing process, 74–75, 125, 243
prayer and surrender, 266–67, 271–72
trusting the process, 249–51

Chinese medicine
acupuncture (also see *acupuncture*), 40, 287
allergies (also see *allergies*), 151, 186–87
bedtime, best time for, 142, 294
emotions and illness (also see *emotions*), 197, 198, 200–201, 207
  joy: heart, 207–208
  fear: kidneys, 212
  anger: liver, 211–12
  grief: lungs, 209
  worry/anxiety: spleen, 210–11
energy, 38–39
energy layers, 105
energy timeline, 86, 171–72
heat in the body, 43, 291, 292
holistic healing, 40, 86, 277, 195
finding the root cause, 37–38, 97, 100, 110–17
fundamental patterns of energy imbalance, 291
imbalances, symptoms, 37–38, 165, 178, 291
jing, 111–12
meridians, 39

moderation, 131, 150–52
organs
    kidneys, 175, 212
    liver, 36–37
    lungs, 174, 206
    pericardium, 296, 297–98
    spleen, 96, 176
    stomach, 137, 139
origins of illness, inner and outer, 200
pulse diagnosis, 109, 110, 290
qi, (also see *qi*) 38–40, 176, 285–86
seasons, exercises, 144, 295-96
smooth movement of energy as goal, 38, 86, 289
stagnation as root of health concerns, 153–54
study of, 32
Taoism, 84, 277
Traditional Chinese Medicine (TCM), 21, 49
Western medicine, intersection, 98
yin and yang (also see *yin and yang*), 84–87, 277
yin and yang organs, 177

cholesterol, 38, 50, 133, 213, 303, 306
chronic illnesses, 44, 103

cleanses, 146, 156–57, 170, 295
cleanse, elimination diet, 147–150
cortisol (see also *fight or flight response*)
breakfast, helping to moderate, 138, 306
fight or flight response, 73, 80
high metabolized cortisol, 304
loneliness, releasing more, 89
oxytocin, 73–74
stress hormone, 72–74, 80, 103

surrender lowering cortisol, 274

D
Dahlke, Rudiger, 172

depression
brain chemistry, 187
chronic inflammation, linked to, 73
good oils/fats, lack of, 306
gluten, affecting, 145
Hashimoto's disease, symptom of, 114
nature helps lessen, 93
organs affecting, 181, 184, 186, 187, 208
physical component, 2nd Key, 97
PTSD, symptom of, 203
serotonin, 105, 185
Triple Burner, aiding in emotional balance, 297

diabetes, 44, 89, 117, 119, 269–70

digestion
antibiotics/medication, effects, 101, 114
best times of day to digest, 293, 294, 306
breastfeeding, 114
cortisol suppresses, 73
chronic health conditions, 113
emotional well-being, affecting, 105, 171
immune system, connected 106, 113, 186
hormones, connected 103, 113
lab tests, 304, 305
Middle Burner, 297
nervous system, connected 104
painkillers causing problems, 102
probiotics and, 301–302
PTSD, symptom of, 203
root cause of health issues, 111, 113–14

Index

season, late summer, 296
serotonin, emotional well-being 105
spleen, 96, 182, 186, 202, 211,

Dirty Genes (Lynch), 112, 116
Dweck, Carol, 236–37

E
ears (also see *kidneys*) 176, 185, 212, 292
Egnew, Thomas, 45
elimination diet, 146, 147–50

emotions (also see *anger, anxiety, fear, grief, joy, PTSD, stress*)
3rd Key, lifestyle and emotional strength, 129
4th Key, listening despite fear, 188
5th Key, emotions and the body, 196–97
acupuncture, emotional effects, 37, 75, 79, 96, 176, 206, 278, 289–90,
balancing, 38, 75,
digestion, affecting, 104–105, 171, 203
emotional component to illness, 197, 198, 200–201, 207
emotional flexibility, 64, 155
gluten, affecting 145–46
heightened, 222
identifying dominant emotions, 207, 234
journal, tracking emotions, 143
moderation, 131
organ-pairings chart, 292
organ systems and emotions, 197, 206–12
origin of illness, emotional imbalance, 43, 105, 106, 123, 200
physical exercise, 154, 211, 222–23 (also see *yoga poses*)
physical pain, 72, 172, 194, 260

qi, 39
stress, 198–200, 213
Triple Burners, balancing, 297

energy (also see *qi*)
Chinese medicine, acupuncture, 32, 38, 40
patterns of energy imbalance, 291
love energy, 76, 87
qi, 39
yin yang component, 84–85

epigenetics, 111
Epstein Barr Virus, 114–15

exercise
3rd and 5th Keys, 222
aerobic exercise, releasing anger, 154, 221
arm exercises, beneficial for the heart, 180
endorphins, releasing, 56, 188, 222
exercise habits, 142, 153, 156
healing process, part of, 306–8
liver detoxification, 211–12
loneliness, social connections, 94
seasonal exercise activities, 144, 295

F
fall season (*lungs*), 144, 156, 180, 292, 295
fasting, 306

fats, health benefits of good fats/oils, 50, 223, 306

fear (also see *kidneys*)
4th Key, distinguishing fear from truth, 164
7th Key, trusting the process, 253–54
breaking the cycle, 221–222
cortisol, 72–74, 80, 103

exercises to process, 204–205
fear to faith, 51, 256, 264–69
fight or flight response, 73, 80, 82, 213, 226
on the hero's journey, 47, 227, 271
KIDNEYS, ruling, 175, 185, 186, 187, 212
listening to the body, 163, 170, 188–89
love, fear blocks, 66-67
navigating fear, 78–84
organ-pairings chart, 292
stressor, 189, 289
surrender, 272, 275

fibromyalgia, 101, 232, 307
fight or flight response (also see *cortisol*)
73, 80, 82, 213, 226

G
gallbladder (also see *anger, liver*)
anger, 211
gallbladder meridian, 107 (ankle), 217 (knee)
liver, partner organ, 36–37, 183, 292
organ pairings chart, 292
spring, ruling season 295
symptoms, 183, 184
time of day, 294
tongue diagnosis, sides represent, 290

genes and genetics, 111–12, 116–17, 136

gluten, (also see *allergies*)
145–46, 148, 149

grief (also see *lungs, emotions*)
depression, 181, 187
symptoms, 174, 202,

LUNGS and immune system, 180–81, 206, 207, 209
in organ-pairings chart, 292
exercises to process, 181, 204–205, 209, 223

grit, 237–38
growth mindset, 236–37

H
Hashimoto's disease, 114, 115
headaches. *See migraines and headaches*
healing, Dr. Shiroko's definition, 46

heart (also see *joy*)
breath work slowing the heartbeat, 82, 84
Chinese medicine, 43, 187
client treatments for heart issues, 120–21, 192–93
Coherence exercise, balancing heart rhythms, 77
fire element, related to, 42–43, 176
heart disease,
    family history, 136
    laughter, preventing, 74
    loneliness, increases, 89
    stress, cause of death, 213
    volunteering, lessens, 91–92
heart meridian, 180
joy, ruling, 207–8
organ-clock time, 293
organ-pairings chart, 292
racing heart, 80, 303
small intestine, partner organ, 179, 295
tongue, 208,

Heart to Heart Medical Center, 32, 313
HeartMath Institute, 64, 77, 91

Index

Hero's journey, 47–48, 51, 66, 227–28, 283

Hormones (also see *Triangle of Wellness*)
acupuncture, balancing, 43, 225
adrenal hormone testing, 108–9, 304
bio-identical hormone therapy, 37, 101
breakfast, protein as stabilizing, 138, 142, 306
cortisol, stress hormone, 72–74, 103
description of, 103
good fats as beneficial, 50, 306
loneliness, negatively affecting, 89
oxytocin, love hormone 13, 73–74, 76
pain, affecting, 102
reasons for imbalance, 103
supplements as beneficial, 104, 223–24
urine hormone testing, 108–9, 110

I
immune system (also see *inflammation, Triangle of Wellness,*)
acupuncture, balancing 43, 206
allergies, and 151, 186–87
Chinese medicine, description 105–7
cortisol, negatively affecting, 73, 89
digestion link, 186
fall, boosting immune system, 292, 295
good fats, beneficial, 50
laughter, strengthening, 74
loneliness, weakens, 89
love and health, 64
LUNGS, regulating, 180, 209, 292
stress, affecting, 73, 102, 106, 214
supplements as supporting, 75, 292, 301
symptoms, 180, 181, 209
thyroid and, 114–15, 187

infections
acupuncture as viable treatment for, 287
chronic imbalances, 112
digestive problems caused by, 114
fire/heat in the body, 43
hidden infections, stool tests revealing, 109, 304
hormones, infections causing imbalance, 103
rashes, infections presenting as, 107
respiratory/sinus infections, 180–81, 206, 235

inflammation, (also see *stress*) 73, 89, 131, 213, 304

intestines. See *small/large intestines*

J
jing (life force energy), 111–12, 150
joy (also see *heart*) 179, 187, 198, 204–205, 207–208, 292

K
Kaptchuk, Ted, 32

kidneys (also see *fear, bones,*)
acupuncture, 289
basic kidney tests, 303
bones, 105, 175, 185, 212
diabetes and kidney failure, 270
ears, 176, 185, 212, 292
fear, ruling, 175, 185, 186, 187, 212
innermost organ, 105, 106
jing, housed in, 111
knees, 175, 178, 185
low energy/fatigue, 176, 185, 187, 294, 295

organ-pairings chart, 292
organ-time clock, 294
symptoms, 178, 185, 187
time of day, 176, 294
winter, season, 185, 292, 295,

knee issues (also see kidneys)
emotions affecting knees, 199, 216–17, 230

L

laughter, healing quality of, 73, 78, 154, 204, 208, 223

large intestines (also see *lungs, grief*)
grief, ruling, 209–10
immune system, connection, 105, 180, 209
LUNGS, partner organ, 180–81, 209
organ-clock time, 293
organ-pairings chart, 292
outermost layer of body's energy, 105–6
rashes, infections presenting as, 107

late summer season (*spleen*), 144, 182, 292
Levine, Peter, 205

liver (also see *anger*)
acupressure to unblock liver qi, 184
allergies, 186–87
anger, ruling, 36–37, 154, 183, 184, 187, 202, 211–12, 295
basic liver testing, 303
blood, regulated/stored by liver, 105, 154, 183
cirrhosis of the liver, 213
exercise/sweating aids balance, 211
eyes, regulating, 176, 211, 292
gall bladder, partner organ, 36, 183

organ-pairings chart, 292
painkillers and liver imbalance, 102
sleep issues, 188
smooth flow of energy, regulating, 183, 207, 211
spring, season, 156–57, 183, 186, 295
stress, 37, 211
symptoms, 36, 183–84, 187, 202,
time of day, 177, 295

love
1st Key, focus on, 13–14, 23, 61–62, 65–66, 125, 234
a healing force, 35, 37, 63–64, 81, 87
heartbreak, love after pain of, 33–35
love and the healing process, 74–75, 125, 243
loving state, cultivating, 67, 80, 221
yin and yang, 87

loneliness, 52, 67, 89–90, 94
Lower Burner (also see *Triple Burner*), 296, 297

lungs (also see *grief, immune system*)
metal, element, 176, 180
fall, season 292
grief, ruling 174, 180, 187, 202, 206, 207, 209, 223
immune system, connection, 180, 209, 292
in organ-clock time, 292
outermost layer of body's energy, 105–6
sleep issues, 188
symptoms, 181
Lynch, Ben, 112, 116

Index

M
magnesium, 300, 301
massage, 98, 119, 184, 212
Maté, Gabor, 215

meridians
blood vessels, nerves, and lymphatic, 289
description of, 39, 176
gallbladder meridian, 217
heart meridian, 180
illness, caused by, 200
liver meridian, 202
lung meridian, 187
organs, pathway of energy, 176, 291
pericardium meridian, 298
qi, travels through meridians, 39, 176, 200, 285–86
small intestine meridian, 208

Middle Burner (also see *Triple Burner*), 296, 297

migraines and headaches
acupuncture, 31, 37, 287–88
anger, expressing as, 202, 211
digestive imbalance, causing, 113
liver imbalance, associated with, 36, 183, 184, 186, 207
nature exposure, reducing, 93
sudden extreme headaches, emergency, 303

moderation, 131–32, 150–53
muscle testing, 191

N
negative thinking as a positive tool, 214–16, 275

Nepo, Mark, 155

nervous system (also see *Triangle of Wellness*)
cortisol, suppressing functions, 73
description of, 104
emotions, connection, 195, 247,
fear, autonomic nervous system response, 80
gut, nervous system, 104–5
methods of calming, 108, 262, 263
parasympathetic nervous system, resetting, 82

O
Omega fatty acids, 301

P
pain
2nd Key and, 102
7th Key and, 256, 257–64
actions and exercises for, 71, 76, 84, 87–88, 91–92, 174, 234
a communication, 44, 166, 170, 258–59
fear, worsening pain, 80
fibromyalgia, chronic pain, 101
laughter, decreasing pain, 74
love, a healing force, 37, 63–64, 87
pain medication, 38, 55, 86, 102, 121–22, 174, 220–21
pain and health, 45–46
physical pain and emotions, 72, 172, 194
stuck energy, causing, 86, 88, 153
trusting the process, 256
understanding your pain, 174
unusual abdominal pain, emergency 303

pericardium, 294, 296, 297–98
post-traumatic stress disorder (PTSD), 79, 202–204, 226, 290
prayer, power of, 266–67
pregnancy issues, 187, 190
probiotics, 301–2
prolotherapy, 230–31
pulse diagnosis (see *Chinese medicine*), 109, 110, 290
pyloric valve, 296, 297

Q
qi, 39–40
anger and rising qi, 211, 218
climatic qi, 292
creation and maintenance of, 38–40, 176, 285–86
emotional release as balancing qi, 204
energy timeline, 171
gu qi, energy of food, 210
illness and blocked qi, 200
kidneys, hold qi, 212
liver qi, 184, 211
lungs, governing, 180, 209
rebellious qi, 182
scattered qi and excitability, 208
stress factors, managing, 196
yin organs, producing, 177

qi gong, 308

R
root cause (also see *Chinese medicine*)
2nd Key, physical, 100, 109–16
actions for finding, 115–16
deeper investigation, 38, 113, 121
digestion as a root cause, 38, 114
emotions and health, 123
energetic root of disease, addressing, 120
four elements to consider, 111–15
lab tests, helping to reveal, 110, 305
origins of illness, inner and outer, 200
symptoms, studying, 107, 175

S
Salleh, M. R., 214
salt, 103, 185, 292, 294
serotonin, 105, 138, 185

sleep
clearing the mind, a method of, 223
emotional well-being, affecting, 129, 213
good sleep hygiene, 108
insomnia and heart/small intestine imbalance, 179
observing sleep patterns, 169
PTSD leading to sleep problems, 203
recommended sleep times, 142, 294–95
sleep apnea, 121
sleep issues and organ imbalance, 188

small intestines (also see *heart, joy*)
heart, partner organ, 179–80, 207-8, 295
joy, ruling, 207–8
organ-clock time, 293
organ-pairings chart, 292

spleen (also see *anxiety, stomach*)
allergies, 186
blood, producing, 96, 154, 176
digestion, ruling, 181, 202
foods benefiting, 183, 211
immune system, as part of, 106
insomnia and, 188

Index

late summer, season, 296
organ-pairings chart, 292
symptoms, 96, 181-82, 187–88
stomach, partner organ 177, 181–82, 292
time of day, 293
worry, ruling, 182, 187, 202, 207, 210

spring season (*liver*), 144, 156–57, 183, 186, 292, 295
stagnation, 86, 132, 153–57, 234, 297

stomach
acupuncture, ulcers, 287
caffeine and stomach health, 138, 210–11
food affecting, 183, 211
late summer, season, 296
spleen, partner organ, 177, 181–82, 292
time of day, 293
worry, stomach connected to, 137, 171, 202, 207, 210

stress (also see *cortisol*)
5th Key, as part of, 198, 213–16
acupuncture, helping to reduce, 287
chronic stress, 85, 213–14
cortisol, stress hormone, 72–73, 74, 103
emotional stress, 198–200, 213
evaluating, 173
fear as a stressor, 189, 289
gallbladder, 183, 184
hormones, as affecting, 103, 129
immune system, as weakening, 105
inflammation, stress increases, 24, 73, 131
kidneys/fear, affecting, 212
liver, deals with stress, 37, 211
pain, causing stress, 102
positive stress, 213

qi, stress affecting balance of, 171, 196
stress management, 136
vitamin D, stress depleting, 301

summer season (*heart*), 179, 182, 292, 295–96
surgery, 99, 114, 119, 120–21
surrender, 252–53, 257, 266–67, 269–75

T
Tao Te Ching, 92, 277
Taoism, 84, 276, 277
thyroid, 114–15, 181, 187, 303
tongue, 179, 208, 292
tongue diagnosis, 110, 290

Triangle of Wellness (see also *hormones, immune system, nervous system*)
2nd Key, as part of, 99, 102
acupuncture and herbs to heal, 43
balance and healing, 101, 102, 107, 124, 126, 234
chronic illness, 102
defining the Triangle of Wellness, 102, 107
healing actions/exercises, 108
lab testing, 108–9
Omega 3 fatty acids, benefiting, 301
pain, affecting, 102
vitamin D, 301

Triple Burner, 294, 296–97

trust
7th Key, as focus of, 43, 254
community support, finding trust, 92
trust in healthcare team, 100, 127

trusting the process, 250–51, 254–55, 256, 264–65

U
Upper Burner, 296–97
urinary bladder, 185, 212, 294, 295, 297

V
vitamin D, 300, 301

W
Wahl, Terry, 305
Web That Has No Weaver **(Kaptchuk),** 32
winter season (*kidneys***),** 144, 156, 185, 292, 294, 295

Y
yin and yang (also see *Chinese medicine*)
Chinese medicine, 84–87, 277
energy, yin and yang component, 84
fundamental of energy imbalance, 291
love, connecting yin and yang, 87
organ-pairs, 177, 179–85, 292
patience and persistence, 229, 230–34, 242

yoga poses, 88, 137, 208, 210, 211, 212, 308

Z
Zazen **meditation,** 217

Meet the Author
Dr. Shiroko Sokitch, MD, FMCP, DABMA

"Healing begins and ends with love."

Dr. Shiroko Sokitch has a reputation as a physician who gets results, and won't stop until she does. Her unparalleled approach to wellness and healing weaves Western science, Chinese medicine, Functional medicine, and open-hearted spirituality into a rare and highly effective new healing modality. After more than 30 years of diligent and determined medical inquiry, research, and practice, Dr. Shiroko is now bringing that potent life-changing healing opportunity to you in this essential book!

Dr. Shiroko's commitment to find answers and alleviate pain began when she was 5 years old, and she never once gave up. Trained as a surgeon, she spent 10 years as an ER doctor while attending school for Chinese medicine. In 1993, she opened Heart to Heart Medical Center in Northern California's Bay Area, fulfilling her dream of creating a center that combined the best of alternative and western medicines. Her life-long quest to save lives evolved over time into a steadfast mission to help people *fully live*, and reach their greatest potential—from the inside out.

With Chinese medicine as the backbone, Dr. Shiroko's nurturing and innovative methods create deep, lasting results. Her unwavering belief that "your body is on your side and it is designed to heal" offers a lifeline to patients who have reached the end of their rope. Few physicians offer the range and breadth of knowledge and expertise that Dr. Shiroko has mastered in her field.

If you would like to learn more about Dr. Shiroko,
including current online webinars and summits,
visit her website at: http://hearttoheartmedicalcenter.com

You can also follow her:
Facebook: www.facebook.com/shiroko
Twitter: @DrShiroko

Made in the USA
Las Vegas, NV
16 May 2021

22945136R00189